WAKE UP

Miracles

Miracles of Healing From Around the World

Edited by
Steven E Schmitt

FIRST EDITION

*See the Miracles
in Everything.
♡ Jamie Clay*

Wake Up Inc
California

Text in Minion Pro, Helvetica Neue, and Raleway.

First Edition, 2020, manufactured in USA
1 2 3 4 5 6 7 8 9 10 CS 25 24 23 22 21 20

All stories, photographs, and author biographical details, in this edition, are reproduced by kind permission of the authors.

All stories were copy edited by Jennifer Blakeslee Peterson.

ISBN-13: 978-0-9994978-9-0 (Paperback)

Additional copies and bulk purchases can be made by contacting:

Steven E Schmitt
Wake Up Inc
PO Box 4251,
Westminster, CA, 92684

www.bestsellerguru.com

Disclaimer:

This Book contains information by various authors that is intended as help and general advice on wellness and health issues. Always consult your doctor for your individual needs. Before beginning any new exercise program it is recommended that you seek medical advice from your personal physician. Any story in this Anthology is not intended to be a substitute for the medical advice of a licensed physician. Wake Up Inc, does not accept any liability as a consequence of following directions or instructions or advice contained in these stories. The reader should consult with their doctor in any matters relating to his/her health.

CONTENTS

INTRODUCTION

Welcome to *Wake Up: Miracles of Healing From Around the World*, a collection of perspectives from a variety of chiropractors, alternative medicine practitioners, therapists, and other professionals, specifically conceived and designed to give you, the reader, as wide a range of unique perspectives on miracles. If you are reading this book, it is meant to be. Essentially, this is a practical workbook about how these authors from around the world have encountered miracles that have altered the course of their lives and those of their patients. We believe this book will provide a comprehensive insight into how miracles are accessible to anyone. In fact, I guarantee that there is literally something for everyone, from stories rooted in unexpected joy, overcoming obstacles and tragedy, and finding the silver linings to share with readers.

Each author, at the end of his or her story, has a personal biography with contact information. We encourage you to take full advantage of this opportunity to reach out to any author of your choice for further information and personal coaching. I would also like to take this opportunity to thank my fellow authors for the excellent work they perform all over the world. It is genuinely awe-inspiring to see the writing of so many dynamic individuals gathered in one place to share their unique messages, secrets, and stories. While you read this book, keep in mind that you also have the capacity within yourself to achieve resilience by being open to all possibilities!

Steven E Schmitt,
Laguna Beach, CA, 2020

WAKE UP

Miracles

THE MIRACLE OF SELF HEALING

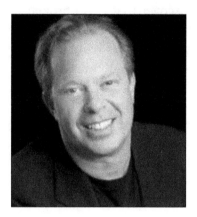

Dr. Joe Dispenza

In order for some of us to wake up, we sometimes need a wake-up call. In 1986, I got the call. On a beautiful Southern California day in April, I had the privilege of being run over by an SUV in a Palm Springs triathlon. That moment changed my life and started me on this whole journey. I was 23 at the time, with a relatively new chiropractic practice in La Jolla, California, and I'd trained hard for this triathlon for months.

I had finished the swimming segment and was in the biking portion of the race when it happened. I was coming up to a tricky turn where I knew we'd be merging with traffic. A police officer, with his back to the oncoming cars, waved me on to turn right and follow the course. Since I was fully exerting myself and focused on the race, I never took my eyes off of him. As I passed two cyclists on that particular corner, a red four-wheel-drive Bronco going about 55 miles an hour slammed into my bike from behind. The next thing I knew, I was catapulted up into the air, then I landed squarely on my backside. Because of the speed of the vehicle and the slow reflexes of the elderly woman

3

driving the Bronco, the SUV kept coming toward me, and I was soon reunited with its bumper. I quickly grabbed the bumper in order to avoid being run over and to stop my body from passing between metal and asphalt. So I was dragged down the road a bit before the driver realized what was happening. When she finally did abruptly stop, I tumbled out of control for about 20 yards.

I would soon discover that I had broken six vertebrae: I had compression fractures in thoracic 8, 9, 10, 11, and 12, and lumbar 1 (ranging from my shoulder blades to my kidneys). The vertebrae in the spine are stacked like individual blocks, and when I hit the ground with that kind of force, they collapsed and compressed from the impact. The eighth thoracic vertebra, the top segment that I broke, was more than 60 percent collapsed, and the circular arch that contained and protected the spinal cord was broken and pushed together in a pretzel-like shape. When a vertebra compresses and fractures, the bone has to go somewhere. In my case, a large volume of shattered fragments went back toward my spinal cord. It was definitely not a good picture.

As if I were in a bad dream gone rogue, I woke up the next morning with a host of neurological symptoms, including several different types of pain, different degrees of numbness, tingling, and some loss of feeling in my legs, and some sobering difficulties in controlling my movements.

So after I had all the blood tests, x-rays, CAT scans, and MRIs at the hospital, the orthopedic surgeon showed me the results and somberly delivered the news: In order to contain the bone fragments that were now on my spinal cord, I needed surgery to implant a Harrington rod. That would mean cutting out the back parts of the vertebrae from two to three segments above and below the fractures and then screwing and clamping two 12-inch stainless steel rods along both sides of my spinal column. Then they'd scrape some fragments off my hip bone and paste them over the rods. It would be major surgery, but it would mean I'd at least have a chance to walk again. Even so, I knew I'd probably still be somewhat disabled, and I'd have to live with chronic pain for the rest of my life. Needless to say, I didn't like that option.

But if I chose not to have the surgery, paralysis seemed certain. The best neurologist in the Palm Springs area, who concurred with the first surgeon's opinion, told me that he knew of no other patient in the United States in my condition who had refused it. The impact of the accident had compressed my T-8 vertebra into a wedge shape that would prevent my spine from being able to bear the weight of my body if I were to stand up. My backbone would collapse, pushing those shattered bits of the vertebra deep into my spinal cord, causing instant paralysis from my chest down. That was hardly an attractive option, either.

Maybe I was just young and bold at that time in my life, but I decided against the medical model and the expert recommendations. I believe that there's an intelligence, an invisible consciousness, within each of us that's the giver of life. It supports, maintains, protects, and heals us every moment. It creates almost 100 trillion specialized cells (starting from only two), it keeps our hearts beating hundreds of thousands of times per day, and it can organize hundreds of thousands of chemical reactions in a single cell in every second—among many other amazing functions. I reasoned at the time that if this intelligence was real and if it willfully, mindfully, and lovingly had such amazing abilities, maybe I could take my attention off my external world and begin to go within and connect with it—developing a relationship with it.

But while I intellectually understood that the body often has the capacity to heal itself, now I had to apply every bit of philosophy that I knew in order to take that knowledge to the next level and beyond, to create a true experience with healing. And since I wasn't going anywhere or I wasn't doing anything except lying face down, I decided on two things. First, every day I would put all of my conscious attention on this intelligence within me and give it a plan, a template, a vision, with very specific orders, and then I would surrender my healing to this greater mind that has unlimited power, allowing it to do the healing for me. And second, I wouldn't let any thought slip by my awareness that I didn't want to experience.

At nine and a half weeks after the accident, I got up and walked back into my life—without having any body cast or any surgeries. I had reached full recovery. I started seeing patients again at ten weeks and was back to training and lifting weights again, while continuing my rehabilitation at twelve weeks. I discovered that I was the placebo. And now, almost 30 years after the accident, I can honestly say that I've hardly ever had back pain since.

About the Author

Dr. Joe Dispenza, PhD.

Dr. Dispenza is an international lecturer, researcher, corporate consultant, author, and educator who has been invited to speak in more than 33 countries on six continents. As a lecturer and educator, he is driven by the conviction that each of us has the potential for greatness and unlimited abilities. In his easy-to-understand, encouraging, and compassionate style, he has educated thousands of people, detailing how they can rewire their brains and recondition their bodies to make lasting changes.

In addition to offering a variety of online courses and teleclasses, he has personally taught three-day Progressive Workshops, five-day Advanced Workshops, and seven-day Week Long Advanced Retreats in the U.S. and abroad. Starting in 2018, his workshops became week-long offerings, and the content of the progressive workshops became available online. (To learn more, please visit the events section at: www.drjoedispenza.com).

Dr. Joe is also a faculty member at Quantum University in Honolulu, Hawaii; the Omega Institute for Holistic Studies in Rhinebeck, New York; and Kripalu Center for Yoga and Health in Stockbridge, Massachusetts. He's also an invited chair of the research committee at Life University in Atlanta, Georgia.

As a researcher, Dr. Joe's passion can be found at the intersection of the latest findings from the fields of neuroscience, epigenetics, and quantum physics to explore the science behind spontaneous remissions. He uses that knowledge to help people heal themselves of illnesses, chronic conditions, and even terminal diseases so they can enjoy a more fulfilled and happy life, as well as evolve their consciousness. At his advanced workshops around the world, he has partnered with other scientists to perform extensive research on the effects of meditation, including epigenetic testing, brain mapping with electroencephalograms (EEGs), and individual energy field testing with a gas discharged visualization (GDV) machine. His research also includes measuring both heart coherence with HeartMath monitors and the energy present in the workshop environment before, during, and after events with a GDV Sputnik sensor.

As a corporate consultant, Dr. Joe gives on-site lectures and workshops for businesses and corporations interested in using neuroscientific principles to boost employees' creativity, innovation, productivity, and more. His corporate program also includes private coaching for upper management. Dr. Joe has personally trained and certified a group of more than 70 corporate trainers who teach this model of transformation to companies around the world. He also recently began certifying independent coaches to use his model of change with their own clients.

MIRACLES

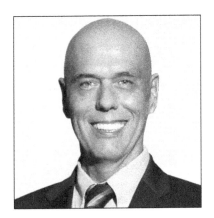

Dr. Paul Drouin

The concept of a "miracle" can have many definitions according to different dictionaries. However, everyone will likely agree that the phrase 'a medical miracle' means "a situation in which a person makes an unexpected recovery despite great odds or a pessimistic prognosis" (Radford, 2006).

Most often these events seem related to the supernatural or paranormal and have an element of faith. The medical world as we know it, based on linear reductionist thinking, can't grasp the nature of these events, so these phenomena are labelled as anecdotal or based on a wrong diagnostic from the start. Conventional medicine doesn't recognize what holistic medicine identifies as spontaneous healing. Rather, the patient (client) receives a diagnosis and prognosis, often of a pessimistic nature, where at best the symptoms can be alleviated but not really cured. In contrast, integrative holistic medicine looks attentively at the nature of these events in an attempt to understand the laws and mechanics that could reproduce such unexpected results.

As long as conventional medicine continues to be defined by the limitations of its linear scientific foundation, healthcare offers an incomplete answer to suffering and the possibility of a healing 'miracle,' so necessary to maintaining the vision of the possibility of a positive healing outcome seems unlikely or impossible.

As I wrote previously, "No one knows the price we are paying for an incomplete medical education (Drouin, 2014). Or maybe now we have some idea with COVID-19, where a global health crisis has almost crashed the world economy. The foundation of medicine must be redefined by a truly scientific model of reality based on quantum physics and neuroscience, sciences that understand and can explain the nature of spontaneous healing and redefine health in terms of full potentiality, rather than disease. Quantum physics redefines modern medicine in a multidimensional reality that not only offers an explanation for these unexpected phenomena but also presents a model for reproducing them. Quantum physics is a science familiar with the so-called impossible or what is strange and rejected by a linear way of thinking. As you read this chapter, I invite you to let down your guard and be open to the possibility of miracles.

Miracles happen every day, every instant. Life itself is a miracle. We need to refine our awareness to recognize, acknowledge, and be grateful for them. In another realm, when we are observing the framework of our natural life, some will recognize supernatural circumstances in which the hand of God was apparent. Others will attribute everything to random circumstances. However, synchronicity will continue to occur in the lives of those who are sensitive to the magic of life or are able to suspend the rational mind.

In my book *Creative Integrative Medicine*, I reveal many synchronistic events that manifested throughout my journey toward establishing Quantum University. When I look back at this outcome, I recognize Quantum University as a miracle that I could never have achieved without the action of a Greater Intelligence. I experience this interplay daily with the Innate Intelligence that underlies everything. One day kayaking in the ocean, I saw turtles and manta rays spiraling around my kayak. This was one of those magic moments we always remember.

The most important of these observations is that miracles happen to those who have some qualities in common: awareness, hope, expectation, faith in the possibility of the seemingly impossible, and acknowledgement of and gratitude for a reality greater than themselves. Miracles are not unique to any culture or religion but are more a set of qualities that can occur in any culture or religion. The technique of Pro-Consciousness Meditation that I offer in the Quantum University curriculum redefines this awareness as a transcendent reality, an innate creative intelligence that is at play in the creative process.

The challenge is that miracles don't occur at the ego level but at the Self level. An effective mediation cultivates a greater Self-awareness and opens the inner vision to the action of subtle energy. One of the first recommendations I make to my student is to practice meditation and, especially, to develop this aptitude for transcendence. As students acquire the knowledge necessary to become competent in holistic medicine, they also acquire vertical knowledge that allows them to grasp the depth of a truly multidimensional medicine.

As you can imagine, I have witnessed the impossible many times during my 45 years of medicine: a patient condemned to have his leg imputed due to gangrene recovered totally; women with breast cancer who were cured; an elderly patient in intensive care diagnosed with a heart attack, kidney failure, and pulmonary embolism who recovered in a week; a young lady free from kidney cancer; a tumor literally dropping from the armpit of a breast cancer client. I could continue for the whole chapter, giving you more details about every story.

But what is most impressive is that I started to observe the same phenomena through my students as they studied a multidimensional medical approach to healing. As they began to acknowledge subtle energy and consciousness and to cultivate a more holistic approach to healing, they also witnessed the possibility of reversing what conventional medicine has declared incurable. These so-called 'miracles' are described in quantum medicine as spontaneous healing, a concept developed in the nineties by Dr. Deepak Chopra. The phenomenon of spontaneous healing is one mysterious healing event that can be understood only through quantum creativity and quantum physics.

Quantum medicine continues to bring more details to our understanding of the mechanics of spontaneous healing, as revealed by quantum physics. Dr. Amit Goswami has once again pushed the boundaries of our comprehension of this phenomenon by adding the core concept of Quantum Creativity. This describes spontaneous healing as having four stages: Preparation, Incubation, Sudden Insight, and Manifestation. For more details, I refer the reader to the book *The Quantum Doctor* (2011), whose content has been further refined in the development of classes that are now part of the curriculum at Quantum University.

The future model of integrative medicine could include training doctors and other healthcare practitioners to blend these two important aspects of healing: the capacity to master the complex flow of scientific information that includes analysis reports and testing, and the power of intention and creativity implied in spontaneous healing. The environment of healing is an ecosystem that surrounds the client's need to be open to the field of all possibilities, where even unexpected results can be manifested.

Would it not be exciting to have access in the medical curricula to the science of spontaneous healing (miracle)?

Creative Integrative Medicine

One of the major realizations I have had regarding this matter of creativity is that we are dealing with a client/patient who is much more than just a diagnosis of disease. Rather, each client is a subject within which an imbalance has manifested and within whom this manifestation can be reversed. The technology of quantum healing resides in the understanding that a client himself or herself is always entangled with the awareness of the practitioner/doctor who plays an important role in guiding their process of healing.

Ideally, the practitioner/doctor will provide the best environment or the optimal conditions for these creative events to occur. When you look closely at these optimal conditions, however, you see that the conventional model of medicine most often fails to provide them. Sometimes the field of natural medicine, too, by reproducing the same model of thinking as conventional medicine, also makes *un faux pas* when setting up a new model for healing.

To make something new happen (healing), we must do something different. Dr. Deepak Chopra, in his book *Quantum Healing* (2015), describes the quantum leap as "a new awareness about the reality in which the client could be caught and has created this deadly condition" (Chopra 1989). This phenomenon is well illustrated in the movie *What the Bleep Do We Know?!* (Chase & Vicente, 2004), adding in the understanding of the emotional chemistry that is associated with it.

It is of vital importance that we identify the ideal conditions in which creativity and spontaneous healing can occur.

Part 1: Preparation – The Importance of Intention in Healing

Before we even touch on the substance of the matter, we must look at the importance of intention in healing. In quantum medicine, the intention of the healer is crucial. The whole process must be based on a proper intention. More precisely, in regard to the entanglement between the observer and the subject (the client), the outcome of healing can be influenced by the belief system and the intention of the practitioner. Many individuals diagnosed with a fatal disease have been able to counteract the negativity and the limited view of conventional medicine, but this requires a lot of character and determination and is not an optimal situation. Most of the time, the patient can only go as far as the perspective imposed by the mainstream.

Quantum healing, when it is really understood, makes the doctor or practitioner realize that they are not at the center of this event (this probably reminds you of Copernicus) but that the client or patient, grounded in the fundamental reality of consciousness healing, is. I am grateful to my clients and patients who have revealed to me the infinite possibilities of healing—from seemingly small to fatal conditions.

After I had been practicing homeopathy for a few years as

part of my integrative medical practice, a man came to consult with me for a difficult problem. A diagnosed diabetic for many years, he had developed a very bad lesion on one of his feet. This lesion was not healing even though he was receiving all of the standard medical attention available, with intensive care of the infected area. After the orthopedic surgeon advised him that the next step would be amputation, he followed the advice of his friends and came to visit me. I listened attentively to his story and suggested some typical homeopathy suitable for his condition. A few weeks later, the client came back for a consult and his foot was no longer at risk for amputation.

Intention is central to quantum healing and, as we have just seen, we may assume that the common intention of any system of healing is to heal. Intention, to be working at its best, cannot be diluted by any other agenda except an act of compassion with detachment. The quality of listening and the relationship with the client is essential in achieving an environment that supports the slowing down of the vital body, using the most suitable complementary modalities or technology for the situation.

Another critical aspect, which is just as important, is to slow down the vital body, as Dr. Goswami points out. Creativity will find its way more easily when someone is in a relaxed mode, rather than in a stressed sympathetic mode (dominated by the sympathetic nervous system), where thinking is difficult. This is more often the case when one has to face the verdict of an impressive professional team, often all white-coated. To add even more tension to this scenario, the words chosen are not always the carriers of a healing force. The fatality of a diagnosis doesn't have the effect of a placebo; it has the opposite effect, where the patient has to face a problematic issue.

Creative integrative medicine, in this context, can help by proposing many different modalities with the specific goal of switching the client into a more parasympathetic mode of relaxation (dominated by the parasympathetic nervous system). Meditation and other relaxation techniques such as yoga (certainly a popular one) can be used. Heart rate variability techniques, aromatherapy, herbology, naturopathy, and homeopathy can also support the client with different cocktails that can do more than just provide relaxation. In some cases, they can open the mind to creative healing.

You have probably understood by this time that the goal is to create, from the beginning, an environment that will allow for creativity. Quality of intention, listening, relaxing, and being compassionate, human, and personal will create the space for obtaining a new awareness about the dramatic and conflicted situations in which the client is caught.

Part 2: The Incubation Period

The second part of the quantum creativity process has been described by Dr. Goswami as the incubation period, where the unconscious comes into play. Everyone has experienced an original idea at least once in their life when they least expected it—either in a moment of silence or after a period of relaxation or a good night's sleep. History has revealed to us so many of these anecdotal incidents, from Archimedes to Newton, true or false, but easily accepted by common sense. For the clinician, what is important to remember is that you can't force the process. This is where the frustration comes from because in the usual model of medicine, things are expected to get fixed just by taking a pill.

Recognizing the entanglement between the healer and the healed is crucial, since the limitations of the doctor/practitioner are one with those of the client/patient. We have already touched on this subject, but the unconscious aspect of the client can be tainted by the limited awareness of the doctor. Not surprisingly, many patients have had to walk away from standard treatments to explore other paths of healing for their own survival. Suzanna Markus, who wrote the book *6 Months to Live 10 Years Later: An Extraordinary Healing Journey & Guide to Well Being* (2007), is a living testimony of a breast cancer survivor who courageously transformed a dramatic event in her own healing journey into the realization of her own full potential of a vital life. She did this while walking away from the conventional path.

A common denominator in all of these stories of courageous women is that they truly went on *le chemin le moins fréquenté* (the road less traveled). They had to reinvent their lives after going through a personal growth experience.

Part 3: Sudden Insight

The third phase of quantum creativity is certainly the most fascinating and has been described as the sudden insight, the Aha! moment. In practice, there are as many Aha! experiences as spontaneous healings in the history of medicine. You have already read several such stories in this book, but you should not expect a specific scenario. These are like love stories; even though you have read many of them, none seem the same, and it is always unique and personal for those who experience it.

So no expectations—it happens when it happens, or if it has to happen. The doctor is not in control of it, nor is the client/patient. The most favorable attitude, and what is revealed in all of these testimonies, is a state of acceptance and appreciation for everything. It doesn't mean resignation; it's more of an active gratefulness for what is and what will happen. There is a moment of creativity that comes with the letting go of it or when surrendering to something greater than oneself.

"When vital energy movement is similarly unbalanced and the vital blueprint is faulty, it is time to leap into the supramental and create a new blueprint of the desired vital function" (Goswami 2004, p 238).

"We wait for [the] supramental intelligence to descend and create the same kind of revolution at the feeling level as the creative insight at the mental level does for mental thinking. The next effect of the quantum leap, the revolution, will be the coming into existence of new vital blueprints to help consciousness rebuild [regenerate] the diseased organs and programs for its carrying out of the vital functions" (Goswami 2004, p 243).

Sudden insights come from the supramental. Creative intuitive moments can manifest like grace, leaving the ego on the side and, helped by the right attitude and a positive environment, encouraging the healer-healee relationship. I myself have observed modifications of the morphology of blood in many circumstances when witnessing the phenomena of spontaneous healing. I believe that these moments of creativity are manifesting themselves more often than we realize. Most of the time, the practitioners, either through lack of attention or by ignoring the phenomenon, don't capitalize on the preciousness of this information. But this isn't the only problem here.

Even if a doctor has some knowledge of this event, it may often only signal the beginning of the journey. In some cases, but in my point of view rarely, the event may be so powerful that it will create an instant revolution that will impact the physiology of the individual. However, this is typically just the initial awakening that the practitioner can build upon and help a client with and, through the use of multiple strategies, convert into a definitive healing.

Part 4: Manifestation

After a creative spontaneous event, an awakening occurs that is associated with a profound transformation of awareness and a revolution at the physiological level, such as a genetic shift or even the formation of new brain circuits. This awakening is at the core of emerging sciences known as neuroplasticity and epigenetics. Dr. Joe Dispenza addresses this issue of behavioral changes in his best-selling books, **Breaking the Habit of Being Yourself (2012), Evolve Your Brain** (2007), and Supernatural (2017). Dr. Bruce Lipton, well-known author of The Biology of Belief (2016), reveals that we are masters of our genetic destiny.

Manifestation is probably the most important phase of Quantum Creativity, in which healing is fully established. The awakening (Aha! moment) is sometimes so powerful that quite literally a miracle can happen overnight. But most often this awakening needs to be rooted at the level of the physical body. Based on empirical evidence, I propose that it takes 21 days for definitive healing to be established. During this critical time, the training and skill of the practitioner or doctor is of vital importance and requires careful anchoring strategies. Quantum University provides important information in neurolinguistic programming (NLP), autohypnosis, visualization, and mediation that should be adapted to each individual's specific needs during this transitional period.

Mind-based medicine is yet another way to describe this large field of interest, and without question, it should be taught to the modern doctor. The step of manifestation focuses even more on the client/patient taking an active role, meaning that along with the process, the new awareness produced by a sudden or progressive awakening will bring changes in habits of all types—from thinking to eating. This is often the painful part of the equation. Who wants to listen to it?

In the midst of my medical practice in Canada, I was exposed to all types of desperate situations and sometimes had to weigh in on how motivated the individual was to accept new habits of behavior. I would ask, "Have you had enough of this problem? Are you ready to let go of anything to see this situation disappear?" Surprisingly, the answer was not always affirmative. I realized that we usually would prefer to have it both ways or even die rather than let go of deep-rooted emotions. I also discovered that more advanced strategies were necessary to support the client moving toward personal growth. The old-fashioned way, where the doctor tries to shake up their client, has not worked for a long time.

Colleges of natural medicine and medical universities must embrace the knowledge brought forth by quantum physics, which reveals that beyond matter is a fundamental and transcendent reality of infinite possibilities that can be manifested through this creative process. The modern doctor, as well as any individual motivated to reach their full potential, should be educated and trained in how to tackle this spontaneous power of healing within.

The medicine of the future will be able to acknowledge, through science and technology, the ability to tap into the infinite possibilities brought forth through quantum medicine.

Conclusion

You don't need to be a saint to witness miracles with your clients. The first premise requires that you be humble and assemble all the environmental conditions favorable to the manifestation of a miraculous event, as described in this chapter. You are not at the center of this entanglement with your client, but a greater caring Intelligence is with whom you are intertwined as a co-creator, along with your client. The client plays the major role. Even Jesus, walking one day walking in a village with no faith, couldn't perform any miracles.

A miracle is not a fix, but a transformative event that when you experience it, it changes your life forever through a new awareness and resolves all conditions that you had previously created to manifest this imbalance. Be silent in the Self mode; listen to your client with presence and see the impossible happen in gratitude.

Chasse, B., Vicente, M. (2004). *What the Bleep Do We Know!?* DVD-ROM. ASIN: B0057IGU40

Chopra, D. (1989, 2015). *Quantum Healing: Exploring the Frontiers of Mind/Body Medicine.* New York, NY: Random House Books. ISBN-13: 978-1101884973.

Dispenza, J. (2007). *Evolve Your Brain: The Science of Changing Your Mind.* Deerfield Beach, FL: Health Communications, Inc. ISBN-13: 978-0757307652.

Dispenza, J. (2012). *Breaking the Habit of Being Yourself.* Carlsbad, CA: Hay House Inc. ISBN-13: 978-1401938093

Dispenza, J. (2017). *Becoming Supernatural: How Common People Are Doing the Uncommon.* Carlsbad, CA: Hay House, Inc. ISBN-13: 978-1401953119

Drouin, P. (2014). *Creative Integrative Medicine: A medical doctor's journey toward a new vision for healthcare.* Independently Published, ISBN-13: 978-1075282577.

Goswami, A. (2004, 2011). *The Quantum Doctor: A quantum physicist explains the healing power of integral medicine.* Newburyport MA: Hampton Roads Publishing. ISBN-13: 978-1571746559

Lipton, B. (2016). *The Biology of Belief.* Carlsbad, CA: Hay House, Inc., ISBN-13: 978-1401952471

Markus, S. (2007). *6 Months to Live 10 Years Later: An*

Extraordinary Healing Journey & Guide to Well Being. Open Doorways Press. ISBN-13: 978-9659112715

Radford, B. (2006 July 29). *Medical 'Miracles' Not Supported by Evidence.* Retrieved from https://www.livescience.com/909-medical-miracles-supported-evidence.html

About the Author

Dr. Paul Drouin, M.D.

Dr. Paul Drouin, M.D. is a doctor of natural medicine, professor of integrative medicine, homeopath, acupuncturist, and the founder and president of Quantum University, the world's largest institution of higher learning to provide online degree programs in holistic, alternative, natural, and integrative medicine based on quantum physics. Prior to that, he devoted more than 20 years to private practice as a medical doctor in Canada, exploring both traditional and alternative methods to further his knowledge of curative, preventive, and integrative medicine.

At present, all of Dr. Drouin's energy is dedicated to consolidating his knowledge of naturopathy, acupuncture, homeopathy, quantum physics, and advanced biofeedback into a model of Quantum Integrative Medicine and an expanded medical curriculum incorporating the new quantum model for health and wellness. He is also the author of *Creative Integrative Medicine: A Medical Doctor's Journey toward a New Vision for Healthcare.* (Visit www.drpauldrouin.com/ for more information.)

Dr. Drouin has also explored and practiced many traditions of meditation and contemplation during the last 50 years. He had the privilege of studying the relationship between quantum physics and consciousness with Maharishi Mahesh Yogi and a group of medical doctors in 1978–79 in Switzerland. He has also practiced the art of contemplation through extensive retreats with Christian Monks, was initiated into Kriya Yoga through the lineage of Yogananda and learned the art of giving Light through the Japanese tradition of Sukyo Mahikari. Dr. Drouin also initiated Project Noosphere (www.projectnoosphere.com/) after the death of his grandson Tommy with the intention of gathering 7 million participants from around the world (1% of the world's population) to join the intention, "Heal Yourself, Heal the World."

Contact Information:

Websites:
www.quantumuniversity.com/
www.projectnoosphere.com/

www.drpauldrouin.com/

Email: nai'a@quantumuniversity.com

Social media:
www.facebook.com/pauldrouin/
www.facebook.com/QuantumUniversity/

HEALTH AND
WELLNESS MIRACLES

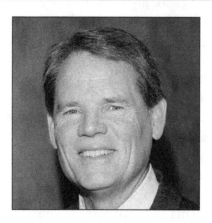

Dr. John W. Brimhall

I have currently been in practice for 48 years. We have developed and use a system of evaluating and treating patients called the *Six Steps to Wellness*. We refer to the classes we teach as "mentoring in miracles." We tell our doctors that if they are not having to discuss the miracles, they see each day in practice, they are missing some of the steps.

My own personal miracle is what started my journey. My father was a building contractor and was from the old school that you worked very hard every day. When I was a young boy, he told me I was going to be a doctor. I asked, "What does that mean?" He handed me a shovel and showed me a footing for an office I was going to dig it by hand. This was Arizona, in the summer, with daytime temperatures over 110 degrees F. At the end of the day, I had dug his trench, had blisters on my hands, a sunburn, was near heat exhaustion, and had a determination to be a doctor—whatever that meant. A side note is we have three sons that also worked for my dad and all have become doctors: an orthopedic surgeon, a chiropractor, and a dentist, with one of the wives a Doctor of Physical Therapy.

In one day and every day since that day, he educated me to get good grades and be a good student. At 18, I was in a car accident that sent me to medical doctors who prescribed pain pills and muscle relaxants. I asked if I should see a chiropractor. They told me never, because they might break my neck. In a few months, most of the acute pain and soreness resolved. I'd still get a catch in my neck or back occasionally, but the doctor said that was to be expected.

At 20, I attended college, taking preprofessional classes to become a dentist. I bent over one day and was unable to stand back up. I was in extreme pain from the waist up and numb from the waist down. I went to the MDs again and they wanted me to take more pain pills and stated I may need back surgery.

That was a scary thought. This time, I was carried into a full spine chiropractor's office, even though the MDs advised against it. The DC (Doctor of Chiropractic) X-rayed and examined me. He explained the accident I had two years previous caused subluxations and fixations in my spine and had also caused soft tissue damage. The symptoms, he said, were covered up with pain pills and muscle relaxants but never corrected. I asked him if I was ever going to be able to walk again and get out of this pain without surgery. He only smiled at me like we were going to see some kind of miracle.

The end of this story was the beginning of my life's journey and work. As I mentioned, they carried me in with severe pain and disability. I walked out of that same office, that same day, without pain and numbness. He told me I needed to become a chiropractor to give back to chiropractic and humanity the gift I had received. It was as if some great force had shown me the life's journey I was to take. My childhood sweetheart and I got married just before our 21st birthday. That same week, we headed to Davenport, Iowa to the Palmer College of Chiropractic. As a wedding gift, another chiropractor (upper cervical/Grostic) gave Claudette her first chiropractic adjustment. She was in the accident with me and was in a previous car accident several years earlier. She had suffered with a constant headache for five years. After her first adjustment, she became pain-free!

We did not understand very much about chiropractic, but we both had miracles and wanted to spend our lives helping others like we had been helped. We came from families with little money, but great work ethics. So, she worked two 40-hour a week jobs at the time and I went to school and worked a job 40 hours a week where I could study on the job and put ourselves through school.

I graduated with honors and relocated to Northern Arizona to practice. God was kind to us, and we began to see miracles early on in practice. In the first few months, one of the more dramatic healings was a Navajo Indian lady, in her sixties, that had been in an auto accident. They told me she was thrown from the car and could walk after the accident but as time went on, she continued to get worse and the medical doctors had not been able to help her. She was now in a wheelchair, had lost bladder and bowel control, and could no longer speak.

After the first chiropractic adjustment, she was sitting up straight in her wheelchair and was talking a mile a minute in Navajo upon her second visit. She even spoke English and told me her bladder and bowel control returned the day after her first adjustment. On the third visit she came in without her wheelchair and was shuffling around on her own. The following visit, she was walking more normally and went on to complete recovery in a couple of months.

That was just the beginning of treating Navajos, Zunis, Hopis and Apaches in Northern Arizona. These people called me their "white medicine man." At first the real Indian medicine men did not like me seeing their people but later there were so many miracles that they treated me like one of their own. It would take a much larger book to relate all that happened with the different tribes. I soon learned I had to be careful because of the miracles they heard about from other tribal members. For instance, an Indian man came in with diabetes and wanted to know if he should go off his insulin after the first adjustment. I had to explain we don't always get miracles and that they needed to work with their medical doctor also with conditions such as his.

There is one experience I feel the need to discuss but am hesitant because of the nature of this miracle. White men of a specific Christian faith, The Church of Jesus Christ of Latter-day Saints brought one of their new members in from about 2 1/2 hours away on the Navajo reservation. The Indian hospital told him he had suffered a stroke. His medicine man told him he was being punished and had evil spirits in him for leaving the traditional church and becoming a Christian.

I did what I always do: examine, x-ray, adjust, and pray. I feel God is my real employer. His face was drooping on one side and he was walking with a limp. I adjusted him, treated him with a percussor, a laser, and sent him back to the Reservation. I did not put the incidences together but within about 24 hours I felt horrible, like a dark force was trying to destroy me. I went to fellow members of my Christian faith, had a priesthood blessing that rebuked any dark force, and called the light of Christ into every fiber of my being. I felt better immediately and thought nothing more about it at the time.

They bought this Indian man back to see me a week later and he was fully recovered. No limp, no facial drooping and no extremity weakness. He felt and looked great! He said he was better by the time they got home from our first visit. He said he had gone to the medicine man the next day to show him that he had been healed by seeing a Christian white medicine man. He told me the medicine man became very angry and said that I had released the curse that had been given him and I had taken it upon myself. That was a very strange experience, but he was totally well and so was I after I had received the spiritual blessing. I have never put this experience in print before, but I feel compelled to do so now. That is the way it happened, step by step.

The next miracle I want to talk about was a lady referred to me for migraines of a 14-year duration. She had been prescribed many different medications and had undergone two surgeries to see if they would help, a hysterectomy and a vagotomy. Nothing helped, she cried, literally. We x-rayed, examined, and adjusted without making any promises. I will tell you I pray a lot about my calling and patients. Helping others like I was helped is more than a job; it feels more like a calling. I told God, "You are sending me all these tough cases. I need all the gifts You have for me and lots of help from You."

Like Mother Theresa said, "With God's help, we can do

almost anything." After the very first adjustment, her headaches disappeared. She was a very thankful person and sent me more migraine sufferers. This was another journey for me in learning. I did not advertise; my patients did that for me. When in full-time practice, we averaged 50 to 70 new patients a month. I had to keep expanding my office, changing offices, and adding staff.

This next migraine patient was expecting the same quick miracle, but it did not happen. I said to her, "What are you talking about, it is not much better? Everyone gets better around here..." This was way too humbling for me! I am trained in spinal adjusting, extremity adjusting, craniosacral and visceral treatment as well. So, I did all I knew, with little improvement.

All the way through school and after, I followed Dr. George Goodheart, who developed Applied Kinesiology (AK). He said, "Besides structural correction of patients, we also had to consider diet/nutritional supplements, as well as emotional stress." We were not taught that in school, so I had a lot to learn. Learning is something I have been doing every day of my life, including today. At that time, I looked up what nutrition might be helpful and gave her the specific supplement recommended. Her migraines left in just a few days, doing the correct adjustments and nutritional support.

When they sent me another migraine patient, I had learned my lesson to give the correct structural care and nutritional support. To my great dismay, she did not respond! I have learned the questions we ask; give us the answers we need. So, I asked the universal intelligence, "What else am I missing? I was impressed to consider more deeply what Dr. Goodheart said, "Correct structure, nutrition and emotions." This was the '70s; it was not cool for a man to be discussing emotions. We were told back then "Big boys don't cry." Some of my medical doctor friends say I am a pathological learner, meaning I am always asking why and wanting to know more and more and more.

In AK, we do muscle testing. I tested her arm muscles and she was very strong. I then said, "I want you to think about what was going on in your life at age 15, when your migraines started." Her muscles went completely weak and she began to cry and weep almost out of control. The technique is to touch them on the forehead on both sides (the frontal eminences) and hold gently there until you feel an equal pulsing. The muscles became strong again and she stopped crying. We repeated this same procedure, starting out with her thinking about the incident, the muscles getting weak, her crying (less and less each subsequent time), me touching the points, her getting strong again and less crying/emotion about five to six times. Her migraine was gone. She went on to complete resolution from more than the headaches. She could function much better in all aspects of her life.

I asked her if she could share with me what happened at age 15. She had been molested by a family member, as had other female members of her family, like sister and cousins, who also had problems like migraines ever since. No one previously had put the pieces of the health puzzle together. We treated several of her family members to great success with this whole person technique of structure, nutrition, and emotional release. These are three of the Six Interferences of the *Six Steps to Wellness* we learned/developed as we saw harder and harder cases. The other three are electromagnetic pollution (like cell phones, 5G, computers, power lines etc.), allergies/sensitivities, and toxic accumulation.

Our motto is "Every Patient, Every Day, The Six Steps to Wellness, starting with Opti-Adrenal." Opti-Adrenal is one of the many synergistic, nutritional, pre-digested, whole food nutraceuticals I have formulated to help balance the body. This nutrient combination balances the hypothalamus-pituitary-adrenal axis and the glands/organs affected from stress, which helps balance structure, nutrition/chemistry, emotions, electromagnetic, and other pollution, as well as assists the body in neutralizing allergies and sensitivities.

A side note on creating miracles is to treat the whole person holistically. If a vault door has six different numbers, you must turn to a specific number, in a specific sequence to get to the gold inside. You cannot skip a number and you cannot say that any of the numbers are more important than the others. In the human however, they may have one or all six interferences and in differing degrees of severity. In other words, you can have near perfect nutrition but be a structural mess and not be well. On the other hand, we see many and most patients that have ALL SIX INTERFERENCES, and all must be corrected with the SIX STEPS TO WELLNESS to get the results desired. We have and do teach how to identify and correct each of the interferences with the 6 Steps.

There is another very important fact you may not be aware of, which is the body has recorded every event that you have ever been involved in and yet you may have no conscious awareness of it. In fact, memories and experiences can be downloaded into you from your family through the DNA. The complete explanation of this would take us into my over 50 years of study, practice, and reading books by Drs. John Bradshaw, Alice Miller, Brené Brown, Paul Pearsall, and lay authors like Louise Hay and Karol Truman, as well at 20 to 30 others. These facts and this information, as well as many others are why we teach seminars, webinars, write books, and send weekly e-mails to thousands of doctors and practitioners around the world. You can access much information from our website at www.brimhall.com.

The miracles we discussed in this chapter all took place in the first 15 years of my practice in Holbrook, Arizona. We started there because we were from a neighboring town a few miles away. In 1986 we moved to Mesa, Arizona, where we had three DCs, a PhD, and a large staff to treat people from around the world.

About the Author

Dr. John W. Brimhall, DC

Dr. John W. Brimhall has lectured with some of the world's greatest health and wellness advocates. He holds two co-patents, as an inventor. He has formulated over 200 nutritional products and is a researcher and consultant for several Nutritional and Laser Companies. He holds a Doctor of Chiropractic from Palmer College of Chiropractic, a B.A. degree in Humanities from New Life College of California, a B.S. degree in Nutrition from Donsbach University, and completed his F.I.A.M.A. (Fellow of the International Academy of Medical Acupuncture). He is a diplomate of the International College of Applied Kinesiology.

Dr. Brimhall's post-graduate work includes motion palpation, Gonstead technique, E.N.T., activator methods, spinal mechanics, Applied Kinesiology, acupuncture, cranial and visceral manipulation, Bio Cranial Technique, spinal rehab, injection techniques and x-ray. He has published works on topics of nutrition trace minerals, toxic metals, cranial and visceral techniques, rib and extremity adjusting, stress, emotional clearing, soft tissue and myofascial release techniques, allergies and sensitivities, and cold laser therapy (LLLT).

Dr. Brimhall is also author of the books entitled, *Solving the Health Puzzle with the Six Steps to Wellness* and *The World's Best Kept Health Secret Revealed, Vol. III.*

Contact Information:
Health Path Products and Seminars
1324 E Treasure Cove Drive
Gilbert, AZ 85234

Telephone: (480) 964-5198
Website: www.brimhall.com

THE MIRACLE THAT HEALED MY SOUL

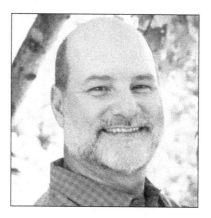

Dr. Patrick K. Porter

Many years ago, two Franciscan friars found themselves shipwrecked. They clung to a small plank of wood, their heads barely above water, as the storm raged around them.

Both monks were devoted to St. Joseph, the spouse of Mary, and so sought his help from Heaven, calling out to him and praying for his assistance.

After a while, the storm abated and the men struggled to get to shore, but the current was strong, and they were too exhausted to make any headway. Once again, they prayed fervently until they saw a radiant figure just ahead of them standing on the water.

The figure greeted them and guided them miraculously to shore. When the pair fell upon the sand, they threw themselves at the feet of the luminous golden being, thanking him for his intervention.

In a small midwestern Catholic church, a seven-year-old boy listens with eyes alight and imagination flowing to a charismatic priest as he recites the Miracle of St. Joseph. The boy fervently accepts every word, while at the same time believing that miracles are a charity delivered by angels to the pious and saintly, and knowing he was neither.

Seventeen years later, in 1985, as an alarm reverberated throughout the plating factory where I worked, I stood over a large tank and pulled a defective metering pump out if it's casing. I glanced at my co-worker, who had his hand on the switch to restart the pump, his eyes wide with worry. I signaled for him to wait a moment and then turned my attention to hooking up the replacement I'd just repaired. I had to move as swiftly as possible, knowing the alarm meant the company was being penalized $197,000 a minute for as long as the waste treatment system was offline. If I didn't get the pump together in short order, it could cost me the only job I'd been able to find.

I was sliding the cover back over the tank when I glanced up at my buddy a second time, letting him know I was finishing up. Just as he flipped the switch, the lid got hung up and a spray of pure sodium bisulfite burst out of the tank and into my unprotected face. I fell back with my eyes shut, raising my hands to my mouth as I coughed and retched. I forced myself onto my feet and sputtered and coughed my way to the closest exit, barely making it out the factory's heavy metal door. Once in the open air, the coughing subsided and I was able to slow my breathing, but my lungs sounded like they were made of Reynolds Wrap. Every time I breathed in, there was a crackling sound. Every time I breathed out, the crackling sound was more pronounced. I spent the rest of the day in the factory's infirmary and was then sent home to rest. My lungs were still burning and crackling with every breath, but my boss and the nurse seemed to think it would be better by morning. I didn't know what to expect but decided to take their word for it. Then, that night, the effects hit me.

I lay in bed with my eyes open, staring at the ceiling. I couldn't sleep. My body was in a severe state of anxiety and stress. This had never happened to me before. I decided to get up. I started reading a book while walking around and doing things. Before I knew it, morning arrived. I had stayed up all night. The next day I went into work and told them what I had experienced. They told me to go home and take some time to rest, assuring me it had nothing to do with the chemicals I had inhaled.

That evening, I went to my parents' house because I couldn't sleep at all. I started acting a bit psychotic. My brain would see and hear things my family didn't and couldn't understand.

The next day I went to a doctor who checked me out and gave me a sleeping pill. I went back to my parents' home and decided to sleep there, assuming I'd get up the next morning feeling rested and my life would return to normal. I closed my eyes with this powerful sedative in my system and slept for only 18 minutes. Once I awoke, I couldn't get back to sleep. This same scenario played out for seven nights, and with each passing day I grew more anxious and upset. My emotions were all over the place. One minute I'd be humming or laughing and the next I'd be in a rage. The anxiety grew unbearable.

My family finally insisted that they take me to the hospital. At first, the doctors believed I had developed Parkinson's. I couldn't write my name. I could barely talk. I was incapable of expressing to the doctors and nurses what I was experiencing. In my head I was thinking clearly, but I couldn't get my body to respond.

After spending two days in the hospital, still not sleeping, they concluded there was something in my bloodstream. They could see it but didn't know what it was. My parents had told them about the factory incident, but they dismissed it, most likely to protect the company that employed many of their friends and neighbors. The doctors agreed that the best course of action would be a blood transfusion, which they scheduled for the next morning.

Before I went to bed, my family came to visit me. My sister told me she was going to send her guardian angels to heal me. I didn't think much of it because I wasn't all that religious at the time. While I attended Mass and did the Rosary every week, I did it more out of obligation than a sense of real calling to be a part of the Catholic faith.

That night, I lay in bed wide awake, listening to the whirring of the HVAC unit outside my window and wondering if I would die before I'd had a chance to live. Suddenly, the room filled with a golden light, but I couldn't make out what it was. I tried to sit up, but my body felt paralyzed. Before my eyes, the light slowly shifted into a form, until I could clearly see the shape of a person, but I couldn't make out any facial features or whether it was any particular gender. As the radiant light filled the hospital room, I felt a calming and loving presence within me, but I still couldn't move, which made me anxious and afraid.

I stared at the light being, my heart pounding, until I heard a gentle voice say simply, "Go to sleep."

In my conscious mind I thought, *I've been trying to sleep for over a week and all I do is sleep for 18 minutes and wake up!*

I was staying at a Seventh Day Adventist hospital in Battle Creek, Michigan, because I was really into health food and they were vegetarian. The hospital didn't allow phones in the rooms, which may seem bizarre to younger readers who all have phones in their pockets. But, back in 1985, there were no cell phones.

I dug around in the bedside drawer for a quarter and then went out to a payphone in the hallway to call my sister. "Shelly," I said, "whatever you just sent me, please don't do it again. It scared the hell out of me."

She paused for a moment. "Patrick," she said. "You're talking."

"Oh, yeah," I said. "I am."

"Earlier today you couldn't speak at all."

My mind raced. She was right. Just hours ago, it had been as if I had a severe case of Parkinson's along with Tourette's because I could only make gibberish sounds and couldn't walk. My body had been shaking and quaking. And now, it was all gone. I was relaxed. My lungs were quiet. I had walked out to the hallway and was speaking to my sister. I was myself again.

So, what happened?" Shelly asked.

"I don't know. There was this golden light, a being actually, that came into my room."

"And?" she asked.

"It told me to go to sleep."

"Then you should do that," she said.

"What?"

"Go to sleep. I told you I would send a guardian angel and I did, so if it said to go to sleep, just go ahead and do that."

"I've tried to go to sleep every night, but I can't."

"Go to sleep this time," she said.

I went back to my room and lay down in my hospital bed. The next memory I have is waking up to the sound of nurses preparing to draw blood. "It's ten-thirty, sleepy head," one of the nurses said. "You really slept in this morning."

I did the math in my head. I'd slept for over 12 hours. When the doctor arrived later that day, he appeared confounded. What they'd seen in my blood the day before had vanished.

When the doctor told me my blood test was clear, I was overjoyed. But they told me that I couldn't leave the hospital until they figured out how they had healed me, which was nonsensical because I'd recovered before they could do any treatment. But I wasn't about to tell them they needn't worry because a golden being had healed me. Although they were a religious bunch, they'd find my story outrageous and label me mentally ill.

They kept me in the hospital for over a month. During that time, I never had a recurrence. I slept soundly every night and spent my days either reading self-help books or laughing and joking with the nurses. The doctor prescribed a daily dose of lithium. I did a little research on lithium and discovered that it was prescribed for chemical imbalances in the brain. I knew there was nothing wrong with my brain, but it was their opinion that I was now too happy, which seemed ludicrous to me at the time, and still does.

That said, I could see it from their perspective. I'd arrived at the hospital angry and somewhat belligerent. My body didn't work and my inability to communicate was intensely frustrating. And, in all honesty, for more than a year prior to the accident, I'd been lost and disillusioned. My life consisted of long swing shifts at work, a couple of classes at Kellogg Community College that I attended half-heartedly, and a lot of partying and late-night pool with the seven other guys who lived in my house. But now my body was back to normal. I was 25 years old. I had a new lease on life. In fact, my whole outlook on life changed after my healing, and I was ready to fulfill my destiny.

So, I took the lithium pill, which they wouldn't let me decline, put it under my tongue, and meditated. When they walked out of the room, I spit it out. I did this for 30 days. Each day they told me they were regulating my lithium levels. On the 30th day they said they had figured out my proper dosage and that as long as I agreed to take lithium for the rest of my life, they would sign off on my release and submit it to the factory that was paying my hospital bill. The company was also paying my house and car payments, so I had to go by their rules. I agreed with a smile.

Upon my release, I told all seven roommates that they needed to find a new place to live and I sold the pool table. Later that week, I received a letter from my employer stating that they took no responsibility for my injuries, but that I was ineligible for work because my body was reacting to something in the factory. They agreed to give me a one-year sabbatical, which meant I would get sick and accident pay for a year. This was another unexpected miracle. It allowed me to move to Phoenix, Arizona, where I took training in Neuro-Linguistic Programming with one of its founders, Dr. Richard Bandler. It also made it possible for me to go back to school and eventually earn my doctorate in Psychology of Christian Counseling.

Most importantly, that miracle set me on an entirely new career path, one that has touched millions of lives, first through the franchise I started and the books I've written, then by way of 2,300 clinics, teaching them new ways of helping their patients deal with stress, and now with the neuro-algorithms and guided visualizations offered on the BrainTap mobile app and through the BrainTap headset. I'd thought the angel, or whatever the being was, had come to heal my body, but in reality, it had been there to heal my soul.

Today, when I think back to the little boy who sat in that church pew so long ago, believing miracles were for others but not for him, I realize that not only are we all worthy of miracles in our lives, we are the miracle in our lives and, thanks to my hospital experience, I've been able to dedicate my life to helping people awaken to this inherent truth.

About the Author

Dr. Patrick K. Porter, PhD

Patrick and his team of scientists and mindfulness experts are leading the way in tech-assisted mindfulness through brainwave entrainment. In the process, they've made BrainTap Technologies a global leader in the personal improvement field. With a library of more than 1000 guided audio programs, BrainTap® allows users to relax, reboot, and revitalize while achieving peak brain performance.

To learn more go to: www.BrainTap.Pro and download the APP as his gift for 15 days and as a bonus his best-selling book, *Thrive in Overdrive, How to Navigate Your Overloaded Lifestyle.*

Contact Information:
Patrick K. Porter, PhD

Chief BrainTap Officer

BrainTap Technology
2861 Trent Road
New Bern, NC 28562

Telephone: (302) 721-6677

www.facebook.com/patrickporterphd/
www.linkedin.com/in/patrickporterphd
www.instagram.com/drpatrickporter/

ACTUALLY, I'M FINE

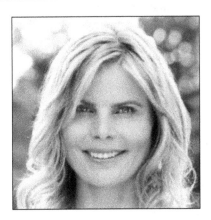

Mariel Hemingway

My story is that I come from an incredible family and an incredible legacy. My grandfather, Ernest Hemingway, was, and remains to be, one of the greatest writers of the twentieth century. While my entire family was creative and intelligent, they were also haunted by mental illness. My grandfather probably would have been diagnosed bipolar had he lived longer or more into this century. I come from seven suicides. My grandfather took his life, his father took his life, and my grandmother Hadley (Ernest's first wife), took her life. My grandmother's father also took his life, along with a great uncle, an uncle, an aunt, and my own sister, Margaux.

I come from this kind of wonderful legacy but also this legacy of suicide, and it has terrified me. Since childhood, I wanted to be this person that was going to survive because I was brought up to believe that I was cursed. They used to call it 'The Hemingway Curse,' and I used to think, "Oh my God, we ARE cursed." My sister, Joan, suffered from schizophrenia. But of course, they didn't know what that was at the time; she was just thought of as an ill-behaved teenager.

My mother had cancer when I was a child of 12 and that scared me. When I was younger, of course I didn't know of other families, so I didn't think my family was different or unwell. I just thought they were who they were. I loved them, and they drank a lot. They self-medicated their pain. Mom had lost her first husband in World War II. They had been married for a hot minute and he was gunned down out of the sky. She never got over that, and I am convinced that this deep heartbreak, coupled with broken dreams pushed deep into her psyche, fueled her cancer later in life.

Every child chooses a role, and I believed that my role was to make everybody better, to fix it all. I became a primary caregiver to my mother when she got cancer and continued to watch my family drink their troubles away, (or at least try to). I knew the alcohol was a bad thing and at about 7 or 8 years of age, I would wake up in the middle of the night to pick up the broken glass strewn about the floor. Once my parents' dinner guests had left, they would fly into a drunken rage and smash bottles and glass everywhere. With thrown wine glasses, bottles, and blood stains on the floor, under the watchful eyes of my cat, I would scrub, imagining that after I cleaned, we could start anew. "Maybe when all of this is gone, we can wake up happier and our pain will have vanished." Thus began a lifetime of thinking I was the "fixer."

After my mother had cancer and my father had a heart attack, I began to realize they were suffering from a lack of communication about who they were and the past they had endured. My father was the son of the greatest writers on the planet and the weight of that legacy was too much for him to bear, especially because he wanted to write. Earnest took his life four months before I was born and when my father was already a grown man. Yet when your father kills himself, no matter your age one thinks, "Wasn't I worthy enough to stick around for?" Whomever you are, when someone close takes his or her life, there is a deep wound of abandonment. Likely, from that moment on, my family began to deteriorate.

Watching the growing sadness and addiction, I chose to become diligent with my health. I was always searching for the healthiest way to live so that I could avoid their distinct kind of pain, which led only to unhappiness. I was desperate to not *go crazy* as I believed was my family destiny. I literally thought that one day I would wake up and be an alcoholic or drug addict, which would send me straight into an institution and I would never know that it had even happened. It felt like a virus I was systematically trying to avoid. I didn't know about which things actually worked to bring me to balance at the time, but that's what I did. My life was all about wondering and experimenting with health habits that would hopefully help me to win my race against destiny.

When I started to make movies at 13 and certainly by the time I acted in Manhattan when I was 16 years old, I was well into my obsession with health and wellness. Well, candidly, it wasn't totally healthy because my habits were so extreme. I tried many different food systems. I've been vegetarian, vegan, macrobiotic, all-fruit, all-fat, no-fat—you name it. I did extreme dieting and exercising for over 20 years, (I even drank organic coffee and fruit only for a year, which as you might imagine, made me hyper and extremely anxious). All during these years I focused on Eastern medicine, acupuncture, herbs, homeopathy, frequency chiropractic (to name a few modalities) and as a result, learned a great deal about health. I became a *groupie* to all the holistic doctors and gurus that I visited. I am grateful to this day for all that I learned from these many doctors and healers as I made myself quite a nuisance to all of them. Those two decades are essential to who I am today… I learned how to meditate, started my yoga practice, opened a yoga studio, figured out a way of eating that was balanced and good for me, and I even began writing books about balanced living.

But I didn't make these changes from a *place* of balance, I chose my journey as a means to survive. I was so terrified that if I didn't make the right choices, I would *lose myself* and not recover. The reason for all the doctors, the gurus, the food plans, and even extreme exercise routines were all external solutions I was grasping for outside of myself. I kept thinking there has to be a person, a diet or an exercise outside myself that was going to cure me.

That leads me to the story about meeting His Holiness, the Dalai Lama. I've seen him before in the United States, but my ex-husband and I went to Dharamshala in India. We've been there several times, but this time we took the entire family. My ex-husband actually had cancer, and this was brought back memories of my mother and childhood, trying to take care of somebody who was sick—repetitive patterns.

One of my sojourns to the enlightened beings that I believed would help me actually led me to India and to a private audience with His Holiness, the Dalai Lama. I'd seen him before in the United States, but this time I was given the opportunity with my ex-husband and some of our friends to go to his home in Dharamshala, India. I had been there several times, but this time we took the entire family including my two daughters, Dree and Langley, who were 14 and 12 at the time.

Meeting the Dalai Lama was amazing, and I was super excited that we were going to actually spend real time with him and the fact that we were going to hear him speak in an intimate surrounding felt like an extraordinary gift for us all. I was with a group of incredible people, heads of huge corporations, magazines, and intellectuals, and each one of them had thought about their questions for His Holiness for months. I, on the other hand, was simply *happy to be there* and wasn't planning on asking him anything. Dharamshala is not a fancy place. The monks preceded him and then he descended the stairs in a very humble manner, no pomp or ceremony. It was actually quite sweet and unusually normal. We sat on cushions and overstuffed chairs, while His Holiness sat in an overstuffed armchair.

The Dalai Lama has me sit down next to him, which was at once exciting and extremely nerve-wracking. For an hour and a half I watched him listen to people from our group. What struck me so powerfully while observing His Holiness listen, is the quote from my grandfather:

"I like to listen. I have learned a great deal from listening carefully. Most people never listen."

These words always moved me, but none more than when I watched His Holiness listen to the group. It wasn't about what he said, it was about how he took everybody in. It was about how he looked people in the eye and how when someone spoke, he saw no one else; he only saw the speaker. It was the most generous act I had ever witnessed.

Periodically through our audience with him, he would look to his right, which was where I was sitting, and he would smile. I would look back at him and smile in glee of his acknowledgment of me and giggle nervously. He would giggle back, and I felt like we were having some unspoken communication with one another – it was surreal. I was entranced watching this extraordinary man. He did say some profound words, but more importantly it was his presence that was extraordinary. His total being and focus in each moment was unparalleled.

After an hour and a half had passed, our time was coming to a close, and as people started to get up, I did as well. I stood up and His Holiness stopped me half stance and he placed his hand on mine. He looked me in the eye and said after a few seconds of silence, "You're okay." In that moment something in me shifted. The journey of my life became more clear and an ongoing fear of existence gently lifted off my shoulders. It was in that miracle moment that I realized I was okay. In fact, I was fine. There was no reason to keep searching outside of myself for healing. This singular and simple event lifted the veil on my external reach and gave me permission to trust my inner-knowing. Over the next couple of months, the realization that solidified in me was/is that *I am my best teacher, my best guru, my best nutritionist, and my best fitness instructor* for me that there could ever be. Ultimately, we are our own healers.

It was the awakening moment of being with His Holiness that opened up the idea that I was the teacher and the person who I needed to heal me. Who knows me better than me and what's right for me? That was when I understood that my message to other people was that we're *all* okay. We all have perfect bodies, minds, and spirits. It doesn't mean that we don't need help, rather, it gives us the means to find the help, which will encourage our inner voice to become stronger. It means that whatever we need for US is inside of us. Our lives are an inner journey, but we keep making it about the outside world. We live in a technical and social media world, one where we buy too many products and we don't take enough time to just be still. All we need to do is listen to somebody we love or admire tell us, "Hey, you deserve to have the greatest life that you want."

Bobby, my current partner of 11 years, has been very instrumental in the journey of self-awareness. He likes to say that we are self-reliant, self-healing, self-sustaining. We have the ability to do great things with our health and wellbeing, and it is in our purview to do all of it. Yet sometimes we don't because we think somebody else has the answer for what makes us tick. We DO have the answers, and I think that is and must be the theme of the next couple of decades for our planet. It's about this understanding of our ability to self-heal once we realize how powerful we really are. Through marketing, external influences, and the power of advertising, we haven't been given permission to understand that we are at the helm of our own wellbeing. This is the gift that the Dalai Lama bestowed onto me years ago: the permission to not search outside myself, but to search inside. All you need to know is that you have permission. Give yourself permission.

About the Author

Mariel Hemingway

Mariel is considered an expert in health—both mental and physical—and is a longtime advocate of personal power, life balance, authenticity, joy, and finding peace of mind through a devoted practice of healthy living. She's both a committed teacher and student in this holistic concentration. In 2014, Mariel co-executive produced the Emmy-nominated *Running from Crazy*, a rich and evocative documentary about the Hemingway family, collaboration with Oprah Winfrey. The film premiered at the Sundance Film Festival and documents her boundless advocacy for mental health awareness, the dignity and rights of people of all circumstance and ability, and her commitment to connecting those of like mind and heart in order to optimize their lives in the best and worst of times.

In May 2015, in alignment with National Mental Health Awareness month, Regan Arts Publishing released two new books including her memoir, *Out Came the Sun* and a young adult targeted diary form project about the journey from surviving to thriving, entitled *Invisible Girl*.

In 2013, Mariel cowrote the book, *Running with Nature*, wherein she and her life partner Bobby Williams share their insights about the import and impact of nutrition, meditation, mindfulness, movement, silence, the beauty of simple living, compassion for self and community, and staying a student of life at all ages. Mariel's best-selling book, *Finding My Balance*, is an honest and inspiring story of her life's journey through the lens of her personal yoga and meditation practices. Her second book, *Mariel Hemingway's Healthy Living from the Inside Out* is a how-to guide to finding a greater sense of balance and meaning through self-empowering techniques and strategies. Her 2009 cookbook, *Mariel's Kitchen*, offers creative gluten and sugar-free recipes and was one of the first to shine the national spotlight on the benefits of this type of diet and lifestyle.

Mariel is a regular keynote speaker at conferences, conventions, and on academic panels where those of like mind and heart gather to educate, engage, entertain, and to enrich each other's experiences. She is also an educator on the power of organic hemp oil, designed to reduce inflammation and stimulate the immune response. Her ongoing focus stays in the health and wellness realm. Recent health, wellness, inspirational, advocacy, and entertainment media profiles include those in *USA Today, LA Times, The Chicago Tribune, The Times* of London, the *Today* and *Dr. Oz* shows, *Huffington Post*/AOL video sites, *Vanity Fair*, the *New York Times, Interview, People*, and *USA Today Best of Magazines*. In 2014, Mariel was the focus of a one-hour interview about her books with Oprah Winfrey on OWN's premiere show, *Super Soul Sunday*.

Contact Information:
Manager Email: melissayamaguchi@mac.com
Manager Telephone: (805) 883-8581

THE DIVINE WAKER-UPPERS

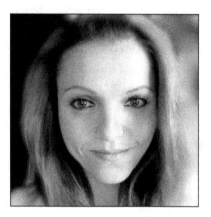

Dr. Evelina V. Sodt

It's all a miracle. All of it, from the infinitesimally small probability of our existence to the families we are born into, environment, chance, and serendipity. And so we float through the world in awe, struggle or blissful oblivion in the name of the miraculous—the human experience of transcendence we call life.

The miraculous was always within reach for me. I didn't grow up with fairies or elves, but I never had to be convinced, changed, or talked into any of it. My great-grandmother, Valasia, healed people with a special form of prayer. I will never forget her serious demeanor as she drew fire crosses with matches over a bowl of water and prayed semi-silently in Greek until the oil droplets she landed onto the water, told her it was done. There were always people coming in and out seeking healing, and it was all done for free. Although there were many rules around its secrecy—there were covenants and conditions too—I grew up witnessing miracles, while feeling an intense desire to find out how these things worked.

The placebo effect could not describe how infants were

healed, for example. It's not like 2-month-olds experienced the biology of belief and yet, Valasia healed babies all the time. Quantum entanglement? Energy transfer? I saw *Star Wars* when I was in the seventh grade, and I was in awe. The Force was the closest explanation I could relate to.

When people think of miracles, they conjure up scenes of a dying woman, who in the final throes of her last breaths opens her eyes with, "I am healed." Images of angels and the beyond bring light, skies and clouds into focus, followed by life lessons and revelations to be learned. But for those of us looking for the formulaic definition of a miracle, maudlin sentimentality and discontent may lay ahead because every disappointment we bring upon ourselves arrives from the little voices in our heads that want to push and predict outcomes. Nothing and no one ever disappoints, only our expectations do.

It works the other way, too. We conjure up extraordinary everyday miracles via the power of intention; we just have to see them for what they are. How do we do that? By walking into a developed, astrally experienced wish. We must do that with all of our senses. We must feel the ease in our step, the strength in our spirit, see the beauty that surrounds us, smell the sweet aroma of our dreams fulfilled, and taste success with gratitude and humility ...all in the name of service to humanity or those around us. But that is still a boxed expectation of sorts.

The key is to stop qualifying discontent, disease, hardship, and strife—because there are none. These things are simply course-changers; they are roadblocks along the way placed there by our own conscious creation in order to bring us closer to our true ever-evolving purpose. The bigger the purpose you dream up for yourself, the higher the price you would have to pay, and the larger the roadblocks you would have to overcome. If we do not clear these blocks, the obstacles will become larger and scarier until awakening takes place, even if that means crossing over.

Our days on earth are prolonged by claiming our own creative power, taking charge, and by conflict resolution, so that the conflict doesn't have to be resolved in the beyond by the legacy we leave for those around us. Therefore, we must not fear redirection, because it is a great teacher. We must not fear mistakes, because there are none.

Only then will our miracles emerge, simply because every minute of every day holds magic in store and sets off cascades of events that lead to other miracles. Yet the ones we actually remember are those, which materialize in the face of adversity—a mom having a baby after she is told it can't happen, a patient recovering fully after being told that death is imminent, or a woman regaining her health after her doctor tells her that she will suffer for the rest of her life. Just yesterday, I heard from a client who told me that his enlarged aorta has miraculously shrunk. These healings to me are actually less miracles than they are redirected human spirit that has been placed somewhat ungracefully and with a thud onto a quest to prove the doctors wrong. Scary diagnoses create determination, surrender, or both. They rock our core to the point of us wanting to enter a new quantum reality. They shift our focus and wake us up. They summon an unwavering commitment to ourselves and make us transform. When that commitment is promulgated by fear, it will mostly likely sustain for a bit and then fail. But if it's prompted by love and a desire to rise above—for the sake of those around us, important work, purpose, or a worthy goal—it will succeed.

Do you remember the part in *The Matrix* where the Oracle tells Neo not to worry about the vase and his act of looking for the vase topples it over? That is how I feel about doctors' dark, permanent illness predictions—the Divine Waker-Uppers. They are essential and without them, the vase won't fall down. Grim diagnoses start chain reactions in those determined to beat the odds. The Waker-Uppers are the very essence of the determination itself.

Our practice encounters them all the time, and I love working with people who are told that their afflictions are forever. My favorite is the there-is-no-cure-only-maintenance pitch. Nothing is more gratifying than seeing people lose heart disease, autoimmune conditions, chronic pain, or diabetes as a result of a miracle—a quantum leap resulting from a Waker-Upper's draconian push into an abyss our clients are forced to fly over. Nothing is more inspirational than our innate propensity for ascension. And it's not reserved for a special few, it's in all of us. All we need to do is reach for it with imagination, an arsenal of senses, an open heart, and self-discipline.

Einstein said that there are only two ways for us to live our lives: "As though nothing is a miracle, or as though everything is a miracle." I want to share mine because it not only changed the course of my existence, it also gave me openness and surrender. It helped me realize that lacking faith is an insolent act of arrogance more than it is erudition. Extreme extrapolations in both directions (pro- and anti-faith) lead us to the edge of the circle, when the center is where the truth resides.

Almost a decade ago, I was working as a marketing director in the NYC metro area. All of the sudden, my whole life was unsettled, and everything felt off-kilter. The company was being acquired, my husband was dealing with several layoffs in a row, I had a young child stuck in daycare into the night, and I wasn't sleeping. I mean, wide awake, every night, exhausted, tired, and wired. Thoughts spiraled out of control, fears, worries, bleak what-if scenarios, and deep, constant angst permeated my being. I was irritable and anxious. I had perpetual low-grade nausea, completely numb toes, achy knuckles, and couldn't move my hands effectively. Even holding the steering wheel required pushing through some pain. That lasted for a while; I just did soaks and massages and kept going. Rheumatoid arthritis was in my family, I wasn't overweight, and the psoriasis in my hairline wasn't all that extreme. It's all genetic, right? I have had mild skin conditions and eczema my whole life, how bad could it be? I knew that stress made it worse and did my best to keep on going. Most days were fine, but some days were worse than others.

The insomnia was what finally broke me—that's what did it. So I started reading. I read about neurotransmitters, exercise, medications, meditation, aromatherapy, herbs, and dietary changes. I did it all with temporary success until I went to a whole-food, plant-based diet. The changes were stark, quick, and life changing. Everything went away in time – not just the anxiety and insomnia, but also the aches, the psoriasis, the numbness— all of it. It's been almost a decade now. That is a "miracle" on its own, but this is not about that at all.

The real miracle here is in the mind-shifting evolution

that created the healing. It's in taking charge and claiming responsibility. I walked into a different version of myself. I looked for the vase and broke it, then picked up the pieces and fixed it. This didn't feel as incredible as my great-grandmother's healing prayers or as my grandmother's stories of magic that created reality, but maybe it was. This healing spirit of belief was engineered in science, the language my heart wanted to embrace.

Maybe it was easier when people had blind faith; today most don't. We have changed the concept, but if we are speaking about bio-energetic dynamism, NLP, placebo, health psychology, or medical hypnosis, why not consider the notion that creating a new health trajectory via mind shift (based on data) is not only possible, but highly probable? The biological changes that ensue as a result of a positive mental attitude are currently a scientific fact. Moreover, the belief system we belong to has one aim only: to possess us and to create a state of knowing, not hoping, wanting, or wishing. Powerful knowing with conviction, lack of doubt, and unwavering strength propels the spirit into another dimension. Our experiential physical reality (that is really non-physical) follows shortly thereafter.

There are so many stories of miracles—triumphant and happy, grand and filled with hope. Stories of healing and good fortune. Stories of prayer at work. People coming back from cancer and from the dead. Yet until today, I cannot comprehend why I still lack faith on occasion. Does doubt make the heart grow stronger or is it the ultimate saboteur? I see it all around me too, and I feel like it's our connection to the divine that is being tested. And that test once again is brought on by a Divine Waker-Upper, the yang of Doubting Thomas's yin, which is the ultimate balancer, because every action sets off an equal and opposite reaction.

The Divine Waker-Uppers bear faith. Then true belief charts the walk, and as we start walking, the path appears. Our belief system is the wormhole that connects us with manifestation. That is why sometimes I envy those with blind faith. I cannot relate to them, but at the end of the day, this comes either from gullibility or from pure trust in the auto-programmed right course of action that exists in the Universe. These special super-beings are not afraid to make mistakes and know that the very word mistake is a judgement call, and therefore illusory. It does not exist. They also know that the perfect balance coded in and around us is oneness. What we do to others, we do to ourselves. What we give, we receive, what we learn, we teach, and what we see is a reflection of who we are.

And so, as I honor the divine source within every person, my spirit attempts to surrender deeper and deeper to the oneness of the matrix we belong to. It's a quest enveloped in instant karma and miracles. May this Force be with you, and may you know you are a miracle too.

About the Author

Dr. Evelina V. Sodt, PhD

Evelina is a doctor of natural medicine, a whole-food plant-based educator, and a therapist specializing in bioenergetic dynamism as a Gestalt of evolving mind-body connections. She is a practitioner, a consultant, and the author of several books including *Healing Pain, Anxiety, and Inflammation Without Drugs: The Science Behind Natural Medicine*. Dr. Sodt practices both virtually and in Warwick, NY. She lives in Northern New Jersey with her husband, daughter, and a cat named Kingston.

Contact Information:
Email: esodt@ymail.com
Telephone: (973) 668-9090

I DON'T EVEN KNOW HER NAME:
A STORY OF SPONTANEOUS
HEALING BY FAITH

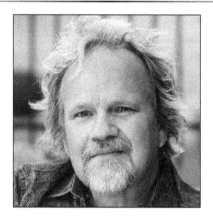

D. Bryan Ferre

Throughout my adult life I have been blessed with a gift that is very special to me, the ability to see and recognize miracles in everyday life. The miracles that bring about peace-of-mind, health, and healing and miracles that align specific circumstances with the right people at the right time. I consider this gift one of my richest blessings.

I was not always this way though. In my youth, I was like most other teenagers, a self-centered rebel always looking for a party or a fight. One day after graduating from high school, I was hiking an old logging trail in a forest not far from my home. I was completely caught up in thoughts about my future. I had not been a good student, so my options were not that great. It was probably the first time in my life I ever stopped to think about where I was going and what I would do when I got there. As these thoughts began to race in my mind, I suddenly realized I was lost—broken and lost. Suddenly, I was overwhelmed with the idea that I had squandered my opportunities and wasted my time in school. Now I was afraid.

I was raised in a good Christian home. I had been taught to pray but had never really tried. Although my parents believed in God, I was not sure. As I walked this beautiful trail, I could hear the sounds of life all around me. The quiet whisper of a distant stream, or the leaves rustling in the wind. I still remember how the world looked and sounded like that day. I decided for the first time in my life to just pray. I got down on my knees and called up to this God I did not know personally. Everything that happened next would change my life forever. I found the light.

A few weeks after this transformative event, I accepted a call to serve as a full-time missionary in New Zealand. I had gone from a child with little to no direction in my life to the ministry. My life as a missionary was filled with amazing experiences with miracles every day. The work was hard at times, but every day was an adventure.

One of my responsibilities as a missionary was to minister to the sick and dying. It was one of the most rewarding and challenging. I spent countless hours at the bedside of people struggling for their last breath. I officiated at funerals and provided comfort to those left behind.

One afternoon, while taking care of the mundane chores of everyday life, I received a phone call from the hospital in Auckland. A young woman had asked the staff to reach out and ask if we could come. The caller indicated I would need to hurry—she did not have much time. I hurried.

I arrived at the hospital around 4:00 in the afternoon, checked in with the front desk, and was given directions to her room. As I pulled back the curtain in her room, I was shocked at the sight. She had a tumor on the back of her head that looked as though it would break the skin at any moment. The tumor was almost as big as her head. I introduced myself and asked her for her name. She could not speak. I sat down next to her bed and I held her hand. She knew that I was there and the spry smile she mustered let me know she was happy I had made it.

After a few minutes, her doctor came into the room. He explained her condition and let me know it would not be long. We spoke for only a few minutes. I understood.

I asked again for her name. This time she whispered, "Please pray for me."

Like so many times before, I laid my hands on her head and began offering a prayer. The words flowed from my mind like so many times before. I asked that her transition would be painless and that her family would be comforted. Then suddenly, almost without any forethought, I uttered the words, "You shall be restored to full health. You will run and not weary and ye shall walk and not faint." Her eyes suddenly burst open. She was shocked. I was shocked. I could not believe I would say such a thing when the obvious end was near. She asked me if I really believed what I said. I responded, "I must."

I sat by her bedside for another hour or so. No words were spoken.

I left the hospital around six. When I got home, I remember thinking to myself, how I could say those things. I intended on a prayer of hope for a peaceful transition, instead I fear I gave her a false hope. These thoughts lingered in my mind for a few days. It really bothered me and over the coming weeks I thought about her often. But soon the memory of that day would fade. I just went back to work.

About three months passed and I received a new assignment. I would be leaving Auckland for a rural town at the far north of the North Island. I packed my bags and headed north. I spent the first day in the new area volunteering at a sheep farm owned by an older man who could not keep up during sheering, one of my favorite volunteer activities. We had been mucking all morning and it was almost lunchtime. As we gathered up our things and headed to the house for lunch and some homemade lemonade, I looked to see a young woman carrying a tray filled with goodies. I was shocked. The woman standing before me was the woman I had prayed for just a few months back. She was happy to see me too.

We sat down on the front porch and talked for over an hour. She explained how the words of my prayer resonated deep within her mind. After I left the hospital that day, she met with her doctors and explained that I had come to heal her body. She told me that the words of the prayer surprised her, but when she asked me if I believed them, she believed them too. She spent one night in the hospital and was released to go home the next day.

The tumor was gone! When she returned to her home in the

north, she immediately got back to work. Her tumor completely vanished. Her final words to me were simply, "Thank you."

I learned some valuable lessons that day that have helped to shape my entire life and career. As we connect with the great oneness of life, we must trust what is. I could have easily ignored the thoughts that filled my mind and inspired me to pray for her complete health, but I didn't. I trusted what is. I also learned the power of love and faith. Faith is the energy emitted by the body in love. Faith is energy that cannot be created or destroyed. Faith is the creative energy that makes all things possible. Fear is energy that is destructive. Fear will destroy everything in its path.

Miracles, such as this spontaneous healing, are not the result of some mystical force in the Universe. They are the result of faith. Believing. This young woman believed in me and I believed in the power of faith to make her whole.

This is how miracles happen.

About the Author

D Bryan Ferre

Bryan is a globally recognized speaker, advocate, and life and executive coach. He is an artist, poet, and author. His work has taken him around the globe, on stage, in churches and synagogues, and more importantly, in the hearts of thousands. Bryan is the author of the forthcoming book The Myth of Knowing: A practical guide to unleash your quantum creativity to achieve your highest ambitions.

Bryan is currently working on a Ph.D. and Doctorate in Natural Medicine at Quantum University in Hawaii. He currently serves as Chief Evangelist for Vivos Therapeutics a company whose global mission is to rid the world of sleep apnea, a pervasive and often misunderstood health condition that affects nearly a billion people worldwide. Bryan's wife, Carrie died from sleep apnea at the age of 44. This unexpected mission has helped heal his heart while helping to save the lives of millions around the world. Bryan is happily remarried and lives with his wife and four children in Utah.

Contact Information:

Bryan Ferre
Pleasant Grove, Utah
801-455-2543
bryan@bryanferre.com
www.bryanferre.com

QUANTUM ENTANGLEMENT, NEUROPLASTICITY, AND HOPE

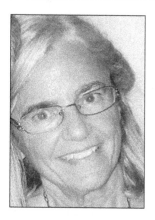

Dr. M. Teri Daunter

Life changes. Accept it. It is what it is. It is this moment that matters. As hard as it may be at times, tell yourself this moment matters, I was rhetorically imparting to a colleague over lunch. We are both healthcare professionals. She is a physician and I am a psychologist. We were discussing the importance of sitting with our patients in their moment of suffering rather than just treating a disease. We both understand the alchemy of presence. You sit and you listen. You wait for them to find their wholeness within themselves and assure them that even in their brokenness there is the sacred.

We discussed the hopelessness of the chronically ill and how lack of hope is a type of violence because it creates a paralysis of will on the individual's mind, since any healing process is initiated as a product of Consciousness. Consciousness is all there is. It is the ground of being. There is nothing but Consciousness. We are a coherent organization of processes and interacting systems initiated from Consciousness. Quantum medicine informs us how energy and communication between the interacting systems can happen instantly without a visible linear pathway. A large quantum sequential jump, or discontinuity, occurs with non-local signals among these dimensions.

My colleague remarked passionately, "I do not believe that as physicians we should give a prognosis to our patients because once they have it, they want to do what the doctor told them will happen." Without realizing, my colleague was discussing quantum entanglement. When a doctor and a patient fail to act as a unit, together they become dysfunctional. Quantum entanglement has yet to become appreciated in healing. In quantum entanglement one "thinks as God thinks," as the Sufis say, in order to bring about a dramatic change in the patient by allowing the patient to plug into the doctor's electrical source and the doctor plugs into the patient to help attune and create a shift in Consciousness for healing.

A bridge is built by calibrating vibrations for a reciprocal flow of energy. Two people become so linked together that the internal state of one determines the possible quantum state in the other. Both doctor and patient extrapolate from these different levels and shift from one perspective, the human, to another, the Divine. This merger creates a resonance because "There is nothing on earth that does not have its correspondence at the super-celestial level, or the Divine Treasury" as Sufi Master Pir Vilayat Inayat Khan instructs.

When one is in touch with one's own inner sovereignty, no pretense is necessary. This authenticity paired with a spoken hopefulness will jumpstart the patient out of limitations and spiritual emptiness. The doctor's awareness then becomes the eyes through which the patient begins to see the physical world. Observation of potential can be transformative because empowering others is the biggest gift we have to give. This unified Consciousness becomes like a pendulum downplaying one level and highlighting another.

I shared with my colleague the same view about the damage that comes with broadcasting a perceived prognosis and provided an experience of a family member who was recently diagnosed with very advanced esophageal cancer. Whenever the physician wanted to give Mark the prognosis, he put up his hand and insisted, "I don't want to know it. This is not the end I can assure you. This is only the beginning. I will survive this." Mark knew at some very deep level that where fear exists, healing cannot. He sensed that if he changed his thinking, he could change his life course—epigenetics at its best. Blood composition controls the genetic response of the cells, and thoughts affect blood composition, which then affect cells.

Mark's cancer ravaged his esophagus and lymph nodes with a very large cancerous tumor perched between his stomach and esophagus. On the seemingly hopeless day of January 24th, an MRI showed no change after intensive chemotherapy and radiation in Mark's grave and very advanced esophageal cancer. On that same day, I segued myself into Mark's healing process and began a crash course with him, remotely, in alternate nostril breathing to aid in bringing both sides of his body into balance, primordial sound meditation to effect the cellular level, and reiki, activities to which Mark had no exposure. No further reliance on machines and drugs, but Consciousness. Then in the spirit of quantum entanglement, I instilled hope by continuously reassuring Mark that once he meditates and treats himself with reiki daily, that his physicians were going to be most surprised when they opened him for surgery. There is no such thing as false hope!

On February 13th, three weeks after the last MRI showed no change in the imaging results, Mark's surgery took place and surprised they were! His medical team found no sign of a tumor, no cancer in his lymph nodes, and only a small section of his esophagus needed to be surgically excised with anastomosis. Mark had eradicated his cancer by partnering with Consciousness through two quantum technologies, meditation and reiki, and shifted the paradigm! He used his mind and hands as a jumper cable to connect the circuitry and rebuild the grid. His pathology report also showed no sign of cancer.

Mark was stronger than his misfortunes. While his physical form took time to make the changes, his mind changed instantly and envisaged the direction in which it needed to go and coach the body. Mark made changes in neural pathways due to changes in his thinking and behavior – neuroplasticity in action! I recall Mark saying to me regarding the quantum energy healing modalities, "What did I have to lose!?" He said he felt empowered to be able to participate in his own healing "…and I honestly believe I could feel changes taking place in my body every time I meditated and performed reiki!"

These felt "shifts" were the clustering of atoms, as a result of his mind's intentions, which resulted in increased levels of energy vibrating within Mark's system. These shifts activated throughout the system began to create new connections for Mark, throwing off old negative imprints and creating new neural pathways. These higher energy flows created a reorganization, since the new patterns cannot be contained in the old structure.

Meditation became Mark's microscope for inner exploration. In this transcendent state, Mark became capable of profound change. He became pro-active and receptive. He became the causal agent of motion. He listened to his inner voice and refused to live in the straightjacket conventional assumptions surrounding his medical condition because he realized there was a dangerous blindness in accepting the prevailing view of society and that of the conventional medical community. This inner pollution is the collective disease of our planet. Being in the here and now transmutes the status quo. This moment matters! The more he meditated, the more he saw the limitations of the conventional conditioned mind. He modified, abandoned, and transcended existing concepts.

Mark's mind became the artist that produced his wholeness. He walked through the doorway of his own integrity to support his healing with determination and perseverance. He was relentless in becoming self-active and self-sufficient. He refused to be reduced into a corporeal entity and absorb the psychotic limiting interpretations surrounding his condition imposed upon him by the dominant medical view. He knew he had super-sensible ideas of his own beyond the duality of psyche and soma. Self-determination, not external compulsion, is an idea that anticipates.

Mark played all the notes in his orchestra and brought about healing out of his chaos. He stopped outward gaze for direction and discursive chatter and rather chose to draw on cellular potential and tapped into infinite possibilities. He dared to wake up from culture's hypnotic dogma, which renders a person into a trance and is one of disempowerment and limitations.

When Mark actively practiced reiki, an energy based Consciousness hands-on-healing technology that has the capability for tremendous personal healing and transformation, it resulted in major changes in his belief system. He offered that he could actually feel the healing come through the palms of his hands. As I treated Mark with reiki at the University of Michigan Medical Hospital after surgery, I watched the heart monitor go from 87 to a steady 65. As nursing staff watched Mark's monitors from their station, one nurse affirmed, "Look at how relaxed Mark becomes during reiki!" The University of Michigan now readily makes reiki available for those who request it. Mayo Clinic uses reiki as a supportive healing modality to manage pain for patients during hemodialysis. They have seen the outcomes.

A study was done measuring the effect of healing touch on the properties of pH, oxidation-reduction balance, and electric resistance in body fluids. They linked these two factors to biological age only. The biologically determined age of the touch-treated group before treatment was 62. However, after treatment for the same group, the biologically mathematically determined age was 49! Reiki is a doorway into the healing world, but it also gives you greater control over your health and your destiny by opening to the limitless energy around you and channeling this energy through the palms of the hands to shift energy into the body. It is guided by Consciousness to create depth, breadth, and natural healing. It came through Mark's heart in a simple and sincere manner.

The organization of reiki is holographic. In addition to using mind and breath, it also uses symbols as part of the healing process. Each symbol reflects the greater wisdom of the whole. So reiki with the symbols attunes you to a higher vibration. Unfortunately, this healing modality has become adulterated by numerous offshoots springing up, as to make reiki unrecognizable and complex. I taught reiki to Mark in its original simplicity. Reiki heals through stillness and simplicity! Mark gave it his wholehearted attention three times a day and became a bridge for transforming his body one cell at a time. Then he waited in stillness; the waiting was a tuning in, not tuning out. Mark became so lost in the silence, as he sat in a pool of Divine Presence, that he became lost to everything else on Earth. His hands became the conduits for Consciousness! He became the instrument of ultimate artistic sensibility. All one needs is one experiential referent to make sense of reiki and its profound transformative healing energy.

Reiki plugged Mark into the energy dance of the Universe, a power so great that all other powers are a pale shadow beside it. Through reiki, Mark became the expression of the Infinite, the electromagnetic flux field of Universal Mind. The preludes and fugues of Reiki healing are a complex arrangement of Divine Wisdom. I have successfully brought reiki back to its authentic, simplified form and away from the "stamps," twists," or "additions" that so many practitioners have added for financial gain. The simplified form is justly a course in enlightenment.

All healing is a product of Consciousness, and meditation and reiki healing are based on the science of physics, the study of energy directed by Consciousness and intention. They fuel a change in energy. It is a change that you, and only you, can create in yourself. An intention on your part alters the chemistry and energy of your being. Healing is not simply a product of medication and surgery. The latter are helpful symptom resolutions, but they are an incomplete approach that only treats the physical and not the quantum subtle bodies that are the downward manifestations of Consciousness from which all healing is initiated. Healing is a quantum phenomenon. Mark's experience exemplifies how quantum healing through mind, energy, and breath can be converted or transduced into another form. You hold within yourself the transformative and regenerative power to make yourself what you will.

This medical case illustrates how one has the ability to objectify any imbalance with the recognition that the imbalance is the priority of the material body and not Consciousness. With this understanding is how "miracles" take place. If you can just get out of your own way and sit with your physical form in silence and talk to your organs, which store all the memories from our life, you would then achieve deep resonance with every cell and every organ and fascia of your body. Exploiting the unlimited possibilities of meditation and reiki for healing, which are accessible to all and are non-invasive, you can create definitive changes from the cellular level all the way to all the major regulatory mechanisms, i.e., telomere length, inflammation, and cell repair to name a few.

This way, you affect the epigenetic landscape without becoming consumed with genes. You have a pluripotential environment in your body that is very fluid. You can readily affect it—in silence. Sit in silence, talk to your organs, which have a Consciousness of their own. Then, just LISTEN to the voice of silence. The voice of the soul and the voice of silence is the breath! Follow the ins-and-outs of breath. Receive intuition and a knowing of what is needed. When you ask for what you need, there is a response.

Mark refused to settle for a "normal" consciousness. He was not willing to wait for some external power to do the work for which he was responsible. He broke awake from herd mentality, an infantile fixation. Somehow, he knew at a very deep level, without being able to articulate it, that Consciousness lived in the timeless present and was available for his healing. He meditated to prepare himself with an inner readiness so that he could become quiet enough to perceive this deep Source within himself through the reiki work. These two ancient and time-honored systems bring changes, which are safe and inner-directed and without the expense of other healing modalities. These two technologies require no expensive instruments, no invasive procedures nor pharmacological treatments.

Through these technologies, Mark admitted new information, which formed new neural connections, and enlarged his awareness as he leaped forward. He displayed that there is no limit to our Consciousness except those created by our own thinking! Our higher Consciousness has a perennial wisdom not explainable by atomic sensory means. It discloses that spatio-temporal limitations are merely optical illusions! The more he practiced the two technologies, the more he provoked growth and changes in the cellular and molecular structure of his body and the more he formed new neural pathways. Mark knew he was not a robot of medical limitations! He continues to be cancer free.

Hope is restorative and biological. Quantum entanglement

and neuroplasticity offer real hope. Hope and health go hand-in-hand. Something deep inside our cells responds positively when we feel hope. Hope is real and physiological and affects the immune system. People's beliefs about themselves affect their ability to get well. Despair, caused when an individual feels there can be no hope of solving his problem by his own actions, dissipates energy from the bodily storehouse in the brain without conscious direction poisoning all the different cellular groupings of which body organs are composed. On the other hand, hope empowers an individual and replaces the energy funds, as it is the antithesis of despair.

Hope extended to a patient allows the patient to see his issue in a different light, undo the imbalance and create a space for a different form. This discernible link between doctor and patient sets the stage for collaborative work. There is no higher or lower level, no hierarchy between doctor and patient. The movement goes back and forth between the two people to allow for a leap in healing by returning to the starting point, our original level—Oneness—by being together in the collective. Both blend and become one with each other so that the two create an endogenous oscillation of vibration and an intense relational space by synchronizing their nervous systems. It is a unitary experience of two people, doctor and patient, from which limitless healing can take place. It is quantum entanglement enhancing neuroplasticity.

As health care professionals we must not barricade ourselves with an invisible pretentious wall. We need to be open to the alchemy that happens in being together, the transformative chemistry that becomes the spiritual dance of life. My eyes became the eyes through which Mark saw himself, the physical world, and his potential.

We need to shift from a reductionistic intervention of drugs and surgery and move into an integrative quantum approach to health, which broadens the scope of recognizing cellular potential ignited by hope and awareness of our consciousness and empowering and partnering, rather than dismissing, our patients. Miracles are a quantum phenomenon and available to all of us if we dare to wake up and let our embryonic Consciousness evolve from Homo Sapiens to Homo Spiritualis. There is an easier way to live.

About the Author

Dr. M. Teri Daunter

Dr. Daunter is a Quantum Doctor with degrees in both clinical psychology and quantum advanced medicine. She has been in private practice for over 38 years at Family Psychological Services in Michigan. She is the author of *THE SPIRITUAL DANCE OF LIFE: Where Two Worlds Meet*, a meditation CD, *Primordial Sound Meditation*, and a reiki manual for remote long-distance training, coaching, and teacher certification, Reiki: *A Spiritual Technology for Global Change*. All can be purchased directly through Dr. Daunter's clinic by contacting her at drmtdaunter@gmail.com.

She has been a daily meditator for 38 years. Dr. Daunter is a global speaker and has had speaking engagements by invitation only on five out of seven continents. Dr. Daunter is also a very accomplished watercolor artist and has had a solo exhibit with 47 of her paintings. She can be contacted at the address above for anyone interested in learning remotely the sacred journey of healing through reiki and meditation or being certified in reiki to train others. Dr. Daunter welcomes enthusiastically open communication with her on all levels.

Contact Information:
drmtdaunter@gmail.com.

MIRACLES AT WORK

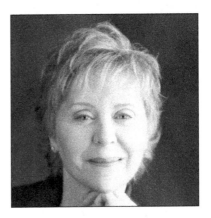

Linda Seagraves

"There are only two ways to live your life. One is as though nothing is a miracle. The other is as though everything is a miracle."

-Albert Einstein

Sharing My Miracle

The fog draped around us like a thick, wet oversized blanket. Swirling images of ghostly figures moving slowly at the surface of the water encircled the boat.

Dad had a passion for fishing in the ocean. With five kids, we took turns going with him and this time my little sister Kathy and I won the prize! We had been in the San Juan Islands northwest of Seattle since Friday afternoon. On Saturday night, dad dropped anchor in a quiet cove off of Friday Harbor. The sky was clear, and a billion stars blinked in the blackened heavens overhead.

Now here we were eight hours later in the middle of a whiteout! "How long can we wait before we have to start back dad?" I asked. "We have to pull anchor by noon in order to make Seattle by nightfall." he replied. "It's going to be tricky navigating the straits without a compass, but we'll do just fine." It hit me like a ton of bricks. The compass was in the bag I had left on the dock.

At high noon, with me lying face down on the bow scouting for submerged rocks, we eased our way out of the cove and into the treacherous waters of the Straits of Juan de Fuca.

Our pace had been slow, yet steady, for over two hours. For most of that time my sister and I sat together on the side bench near dad at the back of the boat. A shift in Kathy's position and soft gasp caused me to glance in her direction. The look of terror is unmistakable, even on the innocent face of a seven-year old. Following her wide-eyed gaze into the distance I saw the hull of a sea-going freighter rising 30 feet into the air. I jumped up and screamed, "DAD!!" as I pointed toward the massive hull bearing down upon us. Quick as a cat, dad gunned the boat to the left and cranked the wheel to the right. We spun around creating a big whirlpool as the propellers dug deep into the water.

Within seconds the freighter was so close we could touch it. No one was breathing. It passed like a phantom ship causing barely a ripple as it sliced through the water. The only sound was the deep, guttural churning of its powerful engines. After what seemed an eternity the ship disappeared into the fog, sucking eerie shapes of swirling grey and white mists in behind it.

We stood motionless, as if suspended in another dimension. Dad finally broke the silence. "We did all right, girls. Thanks for your help." I had to ask one question, "Would they have noticed if they hit us, dad?" "Probably not, Lin; now let's get back on track. Point No Point is our destination."

Another hour passed and once again dad asked me to move to the bow of the boat and listen very carefully for the sound of a bell and look for a buoy. "It should have the words 'Point No Point' painted on the side of it," he said.

I strained to see through the fog, and then closed my eyes and listened. At first, I thought it was my imagination, but then I was sure. It was the sound of a bell dinging as the water rocked the buoy from side to side. I opened my eyes wide, and as if by magic, the buoy appeared bobbing up and down right in front of the boat. On its side, large orange letters spelled out, "Point No Point!" We had made it!

Within minutes the fog began to clear, and we emerged into the bright sunlight. The docks of Point No Point were dead ahead. Behind us stood a dense wall of fog sitting on top of the water like a massive fortress. As we docked the boat several old cronies came down to help us. When dad told them we had traveled 43.2 nautical miles from San Juan Island in dense fog with no compass, they all smiled and one of them whispered, "John, you are one hell of a seaman!" As I listened, I felt as if I had lived a miracle deep within myself.

The Nature of Miracles

What is a miracle?

In my view, a miracle is an extraordinary event or a bewildering impact that transcends known human or natural powers and is ascribed a supernatural cause. How we feel in that moment of dynamic change is an essential component of believing we've experienced a miracle. It is that revealing moment that makes us wakeup blissfully. This unexpected wakeup call helped me look at my life in amazement while I enthusiastically reconfirmed: "I am safe! I am secure! I am alive!"

Is it possible to live every day as an unfolding potential miracle? My answer is yes. You might say, "Okay Linda, that sounds great. But what about those times of chaos and crisis? How do you live the miracle in that mess?"

Mud on My Lens

Good question! In my case "that mess" came in the form of two overwhelming events that pushed me (and my family) to the edge. The first was my divorce and the stark realization that all of a sudden, I was responsible for two pre-teen children and at the same time needed to quickly reestablish myself professionally. The second was the death by suicide of my son-in-law who recently had returned from his second Air Force tour in Iraq. These two things smashed into me and created a human supernova explosion from which I was not sure I would recover. My daughter and her young children, my other daughter and I were in disarray. I experienced for the first time debilitating anxiety leading to feelings of isolation, and yes, even hopelessness. I can assure you I did not experience miracles of any kind for many, many depressing months.

Then one day, similar to coming out of the fog into the sunlight, I saw a glimmer of the reintegration of my family, and myself. Suddenly coming out of that dense fog of sadness felt miraculous to me. Although I had worked on healing myself through meditation, yoga and being out among the trees, my efforts seemed illusive and out of reach until the moment something shifted energetically. Each day began to present small glimmers of hopefulness. I began to notice when someone smiled at me. Soon enough, I cautiously smiled back. I began to feel a little less numb as the edges around me seemed to soften. This momentum was not something I could have triggered. It was when I surrendered to my situation that the miracle came to me—I realized that raising my girls was the greatest joy of my life.

Being A Witness to Miracles

I've had the great pleasure of co-creating miracle quality healing. May I introduce Jerry, Olive and Yvonne?

Jerry is a 49-year-old man who sought help for enuresis. He had seldom had a dry night in forty-nine years. Although the condition had been extensively evaluated during his childhood, it created a level of self-consciousness and stress in his young life that caused him to miss out on the happy experiences of childhood.

As an adult, spending weekends with friends was out-of-the question. His search for a solution continued throughout his adult life. Over the course of seven weekly visits we worked on developing physical awareness and capability using Kegel exercises, hypnotherapy protocols enhancing trust and consistently practicing relaxation techniques. In March of that year, I received the following email:

"Dear Linda, I hope you are well. I thought you'd like to know what success you've helped me achieve. Starting Saturday 1/26, which was the night after I last saw you, I had 30 straight dry nights!! I then had one night not dry, followed by another 15 nights of being dry.

It has felt like a new and welcome world for sure, like a miracle to be honest. Thank you so much for all the care, thought and skill you put forth to help me achieve this lifelong seemingly impossible dream."

Olive is a bright, willowy, and beautiful 37 year-old woman who sought help for feelings of extreme overwhelm causing her to feel so tense that she felt physically "out of her body." Her mind was seldom quiet, so she slept poorly at night, and walked around exhausted during the day. Her work ultimately suffered, and she was not able to keep her job. During this time she was prescribed medication that caused a severe reaction requiring hospitalization.

Olive was tired of it all. Tired of exhaustion. Tired of fuzzy thinking, and tired of dragging through each day in fear and sadness. She wanted to regain her health and experience the energy of being engaged in her life.

Olive and I worked together over the course of 11 sessions. We used gentle physical movements, hypnotherapy protocols helping her to identify stuck areas and move authentically through them. We used imagery to create a healthy, vibrant vision of her desired present and future states. She once said, "If I could release myself and others to live with joy and confidence, I'd feel healed." During our last session she said, "I feel as if I've cleansed my energy field, and I feel in my body for the first time in a long time."

I recently received a note from Olive in which she shared,

"I wouldn't be where I am today without our work together. It saved my life. It helped me evolve and grow into who I am becoming—who I'm meant to be. My return to life feels like a miracle. Thank you!"

Yvonne is a vibrant 98 year-old woman. She was an award-winning driftwood artist who regularly combed ocean beaches and hiked deep forests in search of special wood to "coax into being as art." In recent years her vision had been failing and her health declining, making it difficult for her to move about comfortably. Her mind, however, has the vibrancy of a much younger woman. Her wish is to be able to relax her muscles and brighten her spirits.

I knew I had in my possession the healing protocol for Yvonne —the Healing Lyre. The lyre is a magnificent piece of cherry wood in an oval shape and strung with 48 strings running from end to end on the front of the wood. It is tuned to earth energy of 432 Hz. In music, perfect fifths are known to be the most healing so the notes of B and E, D and A create an enchanting sound while the cherry wood carries the vibrations.

The cherry wood is oval with a smooth back so it can be placed upon the body while the strings are gently strummed. Yvonne was captivated the moment she felt the wood and saw its luster and shape through her clouded vision. During our first session she was a bit concerned. The feeling created by the vibrations in her hands and chest was unfamiliar. Yet, by the end of the session she said, "This feels familiar, natural, and not invasive. It is like I recognize it somehow." As she held the lyre in her lap with it resting gently upon her chest, a smile came to her lips and a quality of unmistakable peacefulness radiated from her face.

Each week Yvonne checks in with me to confirm our next get together. Over the past five weeks I have witnessed her muscles relax and her spirit brighten. I am discovering that the beauty of miracles is ageless.

Practice together?

Do your best to maintain an attitude of effortlessness. Everything you do will be perfectly fine.

Let's experience the breath:

1. Breathe slowly in and out.
2. Notice your body expanding and contracting.
3. Follow three breaths slowly in and out of the body.

Let's relax the shoulders and spine:

1. Allow your shoulders to sink comfortably and let your shoulder blades stabilize and support your upper back.
2. Breathe in allowing the front of your body to relax, open, and expand.
3. Scan your spine slowly from the top of the neck releasing, relaxing and lengthening.
4. Continue to breathe slowly as the muscles relax.

Let's scan the spine and soften the hips, knees, and ankles.

1. Use your breath to scan up and down your spine.
2. Imagine a river flowing down your spine into your hip joints, and then your legs with your knees softening.
3. Flow into your ankles and feet.

Let's take a look at what's out there.

1. Allow your eyes to gaze about without fixing on any particular object or any specific image.
2. Let it be effortless.
3. Release any unnecessary tension.
4. Unlock.
5. Open the door to living each day as an unfolding miracle.

About the Author

Linda Seagraves, MA, SEP, CMS-CHT

Linda Seagraves has decades of training and practical experience in organizational design and development, and, Mind-Body Health. She has helped clients improve their lives in exciting, sometimes surprising ways. These include:
- reducing pain
- lowering blood pressure
- reducing stress
- changing unhealthy habits
- improving communication and relationships

Her education includes an MA in Organizational Development, Clinical Hypnotherapy, Mindfulness-Based Stress Reduction, Trauma Release through Somatic Experiencing, Nature and Forest Therapy, and supportive disciplines such as yoga and qi gong.

An experienced organizational leader, Linda has served as a Marine Corps officer, bank executive and project manager for a Fortune 500 company. Her observations of human behavior and its connection to individual health inspired her to study the mind-body connection.

She began her Mind-Body Health studies at the University of Massachusetts Medical School, Center for Mindfulness in Medicine, Health Care, and Society. For the 12+ years since, she has worked as a stress reduction consultant for organizations and individuals, integrating related techniques such as yoga as a certified instructor and qi gong into her sessions and workshops.

In her stress reduction practice, Linda encountered clients with PTSD and other long-term trauma effects, inspiring her to earn her certificates in Somatic Experiencing (trauma release therapy) from the Somatic Experiencing Trauma Institute, and as a Forest Therapy Guide from the Association of Nature and Forest Therapy.

Linda is a certified clinical medical support hypnotherapist whose hypnotherapy practice is located in the Seattle area.

Contact Information:

To learn more about her practice areas, you may contact her at:
Telephone: 1-425-270-5967
Email: linda@lindaseagraves.com

LIVING BY VISION

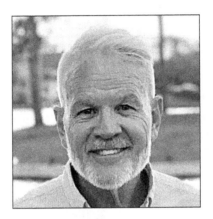

Dr. Jim Hayes

I had chronic low back pain growing up, possibly due to falling two stories off a balcony when I was five years old. Being a typical rambunctious boy, I suffered several concussions, multiple visits to the ER for stitches, and did not reach five feet tall until I was in the eleventh grade. Perhaps my pituitary gland was temporarily affected from the head trauma.

I was always self-sufficient, delivering newspapers from nine years old through my teens, taught myself drums and played in a rock band, had other odd jobs, but had no idea what I wanted to be when I grew up. I started college with no goals and tried three different majors but ended up with a C average after 18 months. I became very frustrated and depressed and was losing interest in college.

Late one night on the university campus, I yelled at the sky and begged God for help and asked Him to give me peace and purpose. I was desperate, but not too hopeful. Within a short time, I began to feel better about myself and was starting to become somewhat optimistic about my future. I had no idea what I was going to do, but over time, interesting events began to occur.

My optometrist said, during my appointment, that he had always liked me and wanted to give me his practice if I became an optometrist. Wow! But what about the reality of making poor grades in all my college science courses so far? But now I had something to shoot for! I enjoyed spending time with him in his office during my summer break, picturing myself as an eye doctor.

Because of my new goal, I left the university and started college over at a Miami Community College. I tried to enroll in Chemistry 101, but they required me to take Remedial Chemistry 100 first. My chemistry professor made chemistry come alive for me. He taught in a wheelchair as he had multiple sclerosis. He smiled a lot and was almost amused at my excitement, in spite of my previous pathetic grades. I worked very hard and to my surprise, I was accepted to Southern College of Optometry in Tennessee.

But, before going to optometry school, I was invited to go camping in Europe by two of my best friends. During the trip, one of them who was in premed asked me if I had ever considered being a medical missionary. Immediately, I became excited at the thought of being a medical missionary.

Bingo!! That was it! The power of a vision.

I came home and told my parents I was going to be a medical missionary; little did I realize, I was already taking premed subjects. I went onto University of Miami and achieved a 3.98 GPA in chemistry, biology and math, and was accepted to the three medical schools in Florida.

I have had the opportunity of being on medical missions and enjoyed practicing family medicine, obstetrics and critical care for 10 years, and then traveling as an emergency physician for 20 years in seven states. My family and I returned to Florida and I work in a trauma center in Jacksonville, Florida.

Mildred

During my private practice, I had a lovely patient in her '60s, whom I shall call Mildred. When she would come in for her appointments for mild hypertension, my office would light up with her joy and enthusiasm. One day while seeing patients in my office, I received a call from the emergency department. Mildred presented there with severe chest pain and was in cardiogenic shock and severe respiratory failure from a myocardial infarction. I saw her immediately and placed her on a ventilator, inserted a cardiac catheter to monitor her cardiac pressures, and administered IV cardiac drips. (This was prior to thrombolytics, "clot busting medicine").

I visited her frequently every day, but she remained in shock. Her kidneys, liver, and even her brain failed, as evidenced by three flatline EEGs. The consulting specialists concurred that her case was terminal.

I knew the inevitable was going to happen to Mildred. After my office hours, I went into the ICU to disconnect her from all life support. There was a gentleman visiting her who introduced himself as a pastor and stated that Mildred had been his personal assistant for many years. I could see the emotion in his eyes. After I examined Mildred, he turned to me and asked, "Do you have the faith to believe Jesus could heal Mildred?" I suddenly felt something stir inside me and found myself saying that I did. The two of us held hands and prayed for her and asked God to heal her… and within several minutes, her vital signs stabilized. I was stunned and made some calls and arranged her to be flown to a large cardiac care center.

Six weeks later, a pleasant woman walked into my office and hugged me. It was Mildred!

Back to Prayer

My lower back pain and stiffness became worse through the years and sometimes when delivering a baby, my back would go into tremendous spasm and pain. At times, I could not run or even lift light objects. One day while driving home from work, I noticed a marquee at a church stating there would be a healing service later that night. My back pain intensified, so I went to the service. The couple leading the healing service asked all doctors to come up to the stage. We were asked to examine people before and after they prayed for healing to verify physical changes that manifested.

I was amazed at the physical healings I saw. There was an elderly woman who came up with an extremely stiff back. A chiropractor on stage said she was his patient and she had been in a body cast for multiple spine fractures after suffering a severe motor vehicle accident. After the couple prayed for her, she could immediately flex her back and started shouting and running around the church! This increased my hopes and I asked if they would pray for me. To my delight, I was immediately able to touch my toes for the first time in years and have been running ever since.

The couple asked me to accompany them two weeks later at a healing service at the Jacksonville Coliseum. I was one of many physicians who examined people before and after prayer. There were about 10,000 in attendance. My wife and I had been married for eight years and were diagnosed as infertile after multiple tests on both of us. We were deemed to not be candidates for in vitro fertilization. The couple prayed for us and proclaimed we would birth a son within one year. I am proud to say his name is Joshua and he is a physician!

The Christmas Eve Miracle

While I was examining a patient in the ER on my night shift, I was summoned to the next room at once. There was a middle-aged man who was unresponsive and had no palpable pulse or respiration. The nurse told me he had come to the ER only complaining of indigestion and that he had no known medical problems.

We commenced chest compressions, I intubated him, and immediately moved him to a resuscitation bay. His heart went through multiple arrythmias, including cardiac arrest, pulseless electrical activity, ventricular fibrillation, and ventricular tachycardia, but it seemed hopeless. Every time I was going to 'call the code' and pronounce him deceased, his heart would pump, and we could feel a pulse. I was silently praying and feeling we should end our lifesaving attempt.

Then, the shock of my career happened. He literally sat up in the bed and tried to pull his endotracheal tube out! The nurses, respiratory therapist, techs, and I kept administering our treatment. I'm sure others on the code team were praying, too. I had never attempted to resuscitate anyone this long before, but he wouldn't give up! This went on for three long hours and it was extremely emotionally draining for the nurses, respiratory therapist, techs, and myself.

The first cardiologist I consulted by phone did not feel that a patient who was resuscitated for this long and went in and out of cardiac arrest would survive the anesthesia and surgery. So, out of desperation, I contacted another of the interventional cardiologists. He agreed to come in immediately on Christmas Eve. The patient had a 99% blockage of his left anterior descending coronary artery, ominously known as "the widow maker." The cardiologist was able to place a stent to open it up and save his heart.

After my shift ended the next morning, I flew to meet my family for our Christmas holiday in Tennessee. When my wife, Heather, picked me up at the airport, I excitedly told her about my Christmas Eve miracle patient. This was not lost on her as she had spent many years working as a critical care respiratory therapist. We joined our family and celebrated Christmas with a fresh reminder of Christ's miracles and how precious life is.

As I returned to work my night shifts and saw new patients, the memory of the Christmas Eve Miracle pushed to the back of my mind. On New Year's Eve, a nurse approached me and said there was a couple in the waiting room asking if I was there. Could it be? I went with her and when I saw them, I recognized our Christmas Eve miracle man, Mike. We hugged. His wife told me she was praying for God to heal him and give her husband a second chance.

Mike, my wife, and I have become friends. His dad rebuilt a vintage pocket watch that I received as a Christmas present. He said, "Thank you for giving me time. I replied, "It is God who gave you time. He just used me to do it."

I have been blessed to have treated thousands of patients and it is a joy to watch miracles happen. If you live by your sight, you will lack vision. If you live by your vision, you will see miracles.

About the Author

Dr. Jim Hayes, MD

Jim is a graduate of University of Miami School of Medicine and is board certified in family, emergency, and age management medicine. As a physician executive, he is a visionary, specializing in changing paradigms concerning disruptive technologies, products, and services. He has 25 years of extensive experience in the network marketing industry developing, training, and managing global sales teams of over 150,000 distributors, marketing a variety of consumer products, as well as hosting conventions. He was a candidate for State Representative of District 20 in Florida in 1996.

Jim and his wife Heather love spending time with family and enjoy taking their children and grandsons to the beach and Disney.

Contact Information.

Email: drjim135@gmail.com
Telephone: 904-392-8462

QUANTUM HEALING WITH LOVE, COMPASSION, AND EMPOWERMENT

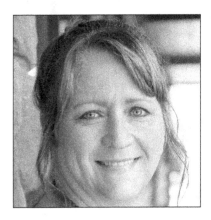

Dr. Vienna Lafrenz

As an integrative medicine doctor, I have the fortunate experience to observe miracles occurring almost every day in my private practice. When I was encouraged to write about the miracles I have witnessed, it was quite hard to identify which ones to share, as there have been so many from which we all can learn from as a society. To bear witness of my clients' transformation from fear and unknown to faith and power of their recovery is almost too much for the naked eye to see, but the resonance of the heart can feel the transformation. It is so palpable to feel the energy emitting from their auric field; you can feel it resonate and combine with yours. I am honored to share with you the magical experiences of clients whose immense bravery, trust, and faith in the healing journey with all its ups and downs, regained their power and health through the entangled relationship we established. I thank my clients who have granted me permission to share their healing journey so others may benefit from their experiences. I am blessed and grateful for their faith and confidence in our combined efforts for their recovery.

Tongue in Cheek

My first miracle story is a 76-year-old female named Jennie, who originally came to see me to "just feel better and have more energy." During her initial assessment, Quantum Biofeedback and TCM tongue assessment revealed the left half of her tongue was paralyzed. She informed me that it had been paralyzed for the last three years from a carotid endarterectomy surgical procedure that "nicked the nerve." Jennie was told she would never regain full function of her tongue and was just resolved to a life of having to modify the texture of her food and experiencing difficulty with clarity of speech. I informed her we would look into what we could do to address that condition, as well as helping her to feel better and have more energy.

After the first session of Quantum Biofeedback, she asked at her next session, "Is it my imagination, or is my tongue getting better?" When I assessed her tongue, there was greater mobility on the left side than previously noted. After three sessions of Quantum Biofeedback, the functionality of her tongue had improved to the point she was able to eat whole foods again without the food pocketing in her cheek. She almost cried when she was able to eat a hamburger for the first time. I informed her that her progression would continue between and after the sessions, as the biofeedback energetically trains the neurological system to attain homeostasis and well being.

Now, when I see her in public and ask to see her tongue, she proudly sticks it out for me (with some sass I might add) to see the whole tongue engaging. She is no longer pocketing her food in her cheek, nor having to modify the texture of her food. Her speech clarity is greatly improved, as she no longer slurs certain words or letters. She once told me, "People don't think I am intoxicated anymore when I speak, as my speech is so much clearer than before."

Entangled Hierarchy for Healing

My second miracle story is two-year-old female named Grace, whose medical history had been tumultuous since the day of her birth. She is a twin, born with a "hole in her heart" and a long history of respiratory conditions related to croup, bacterial and yeast infections, and extensive allergies. Annabelle, her mother, was concerned about the condition of Grace's skin that was covered with a rash containing blisters and pustules that were itchy, bleeding, spreading over her body, and getting worse.

Originally, she was diagnosed with a form of diaper rash by a dermatologist who prescribed six different prescriptions of topical and oral steroids and antihistamines. The dermatologist also prescribed wet wrapping of her skin and "bleach baths" for Grace to soak in each night to clear the skin of bacteria and pustules. The pain Grace experienced from the skin protocol was too much for her mother to bear anymore. The rash spread from her buttocks to her entire body. She experienced bouts of croup that was treated with an intense steroid nebulizer and Albuterol treatments to curb her cough. Additionally, her behavior was out of control at daycare and dance classes, where she was unable to pay attention, hyperactive, demonstrated brain fog, and unruly.

Annabelle contacted me to discuss what we might be able to do for Grace to help her heal, as she was getting worse. She was completing her PhD in Natural Medicine and observed the energetic healing benefits of Quantum Biofeedback and other natural healing modalities provided to clients during her practicum at my clinic. Given her knowledge and experience, she agreed with my suggestion to start with Quantum Biofeedback to identify the root cause of the severe symptoms attributing to Grace's skin condition.

Her initial assessment identified energetic organ and meridian stagnation, adrenal fatigue, presence of candida, yeast, fungus, mold, parasites, tapeworms, bacteria, and extensive food and synthetic allergies, including chlorine, steroids, and sugar. Annabelle implemented all recommendations and suggestions immediately, including discontinuing the bleach baths, steroids, and antihistamines. We implemented a plant-based alkaline nutrition plan devoid of sugars and dairy, allowing some clean and organic meats, increased water consumption, organ and blood detoxification, and avoidance of food and environmental allergens. Her bathing protocol changed to baths with Epsom salts containing pure therapeutic-grade essential oils of lavender and tea tree, followed by jojoba oil for skin support. Annabelle understood the importance of energy and frequencies while performing the nightly routine and consciously infused love and healing frequencies into Grace as she performed this daily routine with her daughter with laughter and joy. We continued the remote Quantum Biofeedback sessions weekly, altering her protocols and plans based on progression of her healing and upgraded her nutrition and food choices.

Within five Quantum Biofeedback sessions, Annabelle reported a significant improvement in Grace's skin health, reduction of pain, and discomfort. She also reported improved energy, sleep, quality and frequency of bowel movements, and increased hydration. Grace responded well to the changes in her nutrition plan and welcomed the fresh fruit and vegetables to the point she would tell on her teachers who would try to offer her any type of sugar, by telling them, "I am not supposed to have sugar."

Her skin condition is back to normal with the rash and blisters completely healed. Grace started to show signs of croup returning with a dry, hacking, and fatiguing cough, which would normally last for five to eight days and through Quantum Biofeedback, was able to resolve it in less than 24 hours. Grace still experiences some skin irritations when eating processed and sugary foods but responds quickly to detoxification and returning back to a normal healthy diet. Annabelle reports she is very obedient and calm and a completely different child.

Annabelle recently took Grace back to the dermatologist who could not believe the improvement in her skin and overall health and vitality.

Planning Her Own Funeral

My third and final story is about a 39-year-old female named Anna who came to me after a surgical procedure following a diagnosis of exploding disc syndrome involving eight burst fractures in the thoracic and lumbar spine. She had surgery on the T9 through L3 vertebral region, utilizing posterior thoracolumbar fusion hardware, which was infected with staph upon surgical entry into her spine. She had to undergo a second surgery to clean out the infection, which required her to have a PICC line for antibiotics. She was in and out of the emergency room following both surgeries due to intense pain, fear of further fractures, and the suture site constantly bursting open and discharging murky yellow fluids. Her surgical wound failed to close due to the staph infection coursing through her body.

Anna's mother brought her to my clinic two months after her second surgery, based on a referral from a close friend who was under my care. Upon her initial assessment, her pain level was a 9/10 consistently and she suffered daily frequent and uncontrollable muscle spasms that would be so severe she would lose urinary control. She walked with a cane or walker for stability and was very guarded and stiff movement patterns. Anna was dependent on her three young girls and her mother for her daily care and mobility.

She was prescribed several pain medications, muscle relaxants, 12 forms of oral and IV antibiotics, and relied heavily on alcohol to help relieve her pain symptoms. She had to sleep in a recliner in an upright position, with pillows positioned around her to pad her against any movements that may initiate a spasm, which affected the quality and quantity of her sleep. Anna had lost four inches in height as a result of her surgical procedures. She reported to me her pain, discomfort, and quality of life was so compromised she and her mother were making arrangements for her funeral and the care of her daughters ages six, seven, and nine, as she did not feel she was going to survive this ordeal.

Initially, we started using weekly training sessions of Quantum Biofeedback to identify energetically what was causing the most stress in the body, mind, and spirit, leading to disease and preventing her recovery. After her first session, Anna reported immediate results in the level and intensity of pain and frequency of debilitating muscle spasms. We incorporated natural remedies to rid her body of the bacteria and toxicity evident in her blood and organs. We cleaned her diet to include fresh whole fruits and vegetables, essential fatty acids, reduction of sugar and alcohol, and implemented natural methods and strategies to manage her pain and muscle spasms.

From the beginning, Anna followed through with all recommendations without question, demonstrating her strive to recover completely so she could raise her kids and regain her quality of life. Within the first four weeks, Anna finally felt she was out of danger of losing her life with a marked increase in mobility, ability to perform some of her self-care activities, and ability to manage her pain and muscle spasms. As a result of the amount and intensity of the prescribed antibiotics, she developed candida, which we addressed utilizing natural interventions to eradicate it, with great success.

Once her surgical wound closed completely, we initiated bodywork utilizing myofascial release and craniosacral therapy to promote greater flexibility in her body and spine. After one session of bodywork, she regained one and half inches in height, confirmed by her surgeon during her post-surgical appointment. Anna was informed by the infectious disease physician that she would be on antibiotics for the rest of her life, as long as the infected hardware remained in her spine.

Within five months from our initial session, she was able to do all her self-care tasks independently, including caring for her children, driving, walking without devices, sleeping in her own bed and performing her own housework. She is off pain medications and muscle relaxants. Anna is back to coaching wrestling, fishing, and horseback riding. She is able to reach her feet to put on her own shoes, squat to put wood in the fire, and is now motivated to quit smoking and lose weight. The medical community expressed their surprise and amazement to the speed and level of recovery she experienced. Her bone density scans indicated sufficient improvement that within a year of her initial surgery, she will be able to have the staph-infected hardware removed from her spine permanently. We added to our goals to attain greater bone density strength and stability and increase overall muscle strength and mobility to have the hardware permanently removed. Anna is a miracle, who readily shares her experiences and knowledge with others who may be dealing with health challenges and obstacles, in order to give back to her community.

In Summary

I would like to share some profound conclusions I have witnessed with clients who get stuck in their physical, mental, psychological, emotional, and spiritual conditions. First and foremost, we need to focus on raising the frequency and vibration within the person in order to promote true healing. We need to identify and resolve emotional, psychological, and physical traumas that may be holding them hostage. Helping them identify self-limiting thoughts, beliefs, and word choices used in their everyday language – both internal and external—is key to their recovery. I have found that most of my clients have difficulty identifying and expressing things they love about themselves. It is imperative we look at the whole person, not just the symptoms, to identify the root cause of the dis-ease that is impacting their health and wellness. Supporting and educating our clients to regain their power in healing themselves is paramount to a lifetime of health and vitality.

During my 30 years of experience in the healthcare industry, I have observed how a person's internal and external feelings and thoughts can hamper functional outcomes and expectations. For example, I was working with a five-star Army General who had a stroke and was receiving rehabilitation in a nursing home. He kept getting angry and frustrated that his body would not cooperate to what he wanted it to do. He repeatedly complained that "his body is no good and is useless." I found the more frustrated he became, the more his body would not respond to the neuro based techniques I was using to facilitate the expected performance.

Finally, I leaned in, looked him squarely in the eyes and asked him to repeat after me, "I love my body and my body loves me back." He scornfully and angrily repeated the phrase, with no apparent regard for the exercise. I patiently asked him to repeat the phrase with love and meaning, to which he sarcastically repeated the phrase. I asked him again to repeat the phrase, but this time with belief and feeling. Tears welled in his eyes, as he repeated the phrase, while breaking down the barriers that held him. This time, when he went to perform the functional task, his body released and easily performed the task required. His expression lit up with disbelief and anticipation at the same time. We repeated the task over and over, until he tired with sheer joy and enthusiasm. He asked if I was a miracle worker, to which I replied, "No, you are the miracle when you believe and love yourself enough to let go of the self-loathing statements and replace them with loving and encouraging beliefs."

To this day, I have found my "I love my body" phrase to help so many of my clients to become more conscious of the words, phrases and unrealistic expectations they create in their everyday lives that prevent them from attaining their limitless possibilities.

About the Author

Dr. Vienna Lafrenz, PhD, IMD

Vienna graduated with her Doctorate and PhD in Integrative Medicine from Quantum University in October 2016. She received certification as a Brain mapping and Neurofeedback Technician in March 2015. Her PhD dissertation focused on the reduction of chronic pain using pulsed therapeutic ultrasound over acupuncture points, demonstrated through brain mapping the clients before and after one treatment, which resulted in a reduction in pain symptoms and resultant changes in the brain. She has specialized knowledge and experience in pain management, craniosacral and myofascial release, heavy metal and organ detoxification, orthopedic conditions, degenerative diseases, autoimmune disorders, bariatrics, lymphedema, cognition, urinary continence, low-vision, and neurological deficits for the past 25 years.

She is internationally certified in Neurodevelopmental Treatment (NDT), Brain mapping and Neurofeedback Specialist, Certified Lymphedema Therapist, Board Certified Health Coach, Certified Chopra Teacher in Ayurveda, and a Biofeedback and Neurofeedback Specialist. Dr. Lafrenz has her own integrative and natural medicine practice in Washington State. She has presented professionally in healthcare settings throughout the United States, universities, and world summits on a wide range of topics.

At her clinic, she offers the following services and modalities to her clients: Quantum Biofeedback (remotely and in person), Gas Discharge Visualization, iridology, hypnotherapy, neurolinguistic programming, emotional freedom technique, heart rate variability, mindfulness meditation and techniques, acupressure, aromatherapy, auriculotherapy, ionic foot detoxification, far-infrared sauna, physical agent modalities, nutritional support, vibrational sound therapy including Tibetan bowls, Himalayan crystal bowls, tuning forks, and sound therapy, various energy and body work strategies including craniosacral, myofascial release, and reiki.

Contact Information:

Dr. Vienna Lafrenz, PhD, IMD, HC, OTR/L
Natural Therapeutics, LLC
Vienna@natural-therapeutics.com
www.natural-therapeutics.com
Cell: (253) 228-0318
Office: (509) 779-0998

READY OR NOT: LIFE IS A CASCADE OF MIRACLES

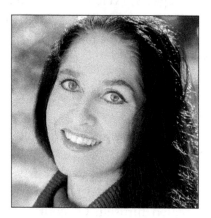

Dr. Manja H. Podratz

We all are born into a human body, yet that alone doesn't mean that upon birth we fully arrive on this earth. Newborns still gaze into the beyond. Their skulls are still soft and the crown chakras wide open. About 18 to 24 months after the body is born, the human ego is also born. Jacques Lacan, the twentieth century psychoanalyst, described the point in time when a toddler recognizes their own image and self-identifies as 'I,' the mirror stage. Up until that moment, we are one and connected with the Source of all creation.

It takes years for our physical bodies to grow up; this vehicle for our ego-identity. We look into a mirror and say, "That's me." It is this "I" identity that separates us from others and creates the illusion of being a unique individual. However, the mere fact that we have grown-up bodies and exclaim our individuality does not automatically imply that we know what the physical body needs or how to be aware of our behavior in ego-mode. More often than not, we take everything for granted: being alive, being healthy, and having a life ahead of us.

It was the year 2000.

"You will have to take about two weeks off. Here, I scheduled the surgery for you at this hospital." To do what? Uterine cancer and a hysterectomy at age 23? "What were my chances, if I'd refuse the procedure?" I heard myself asking, "I don't know. In the 20 years of my practice, I never had a patient refuse a recommended surgery," my gynecologist replied. Wow! "I guess, I will be your first one then. You see, I know with certainty that I will be a mom one day. I still need my uterus. What you offer me here would not heal, only cripple me."

Saying those words was one thing. I felt pretty bold. But after walking out of the doctor's office, I thought, *what now?* I need to figure out how to heal this cancer. My father suggested raw food. He had been diagnosed with prostate cancer a few years earlier and healed himself. Of course, being the young college kid that I was, I had questioned my dad's sanity when he announced that he went raw food vegan. And here I found myself receiving a scary diagnosis and facing decisions with serious consequences.

There had to be a way. As a woman who menstruated every month, renewing the cells in my uterus every month, there had to be a way to influence if those new cells would be healthy or abnormal growth. For too long, I had overburdened my body with junk food, stress, and toxins. So, I started fastening, drinking green clay, and raw juices. I felt my energy levels going up! Following the old teaching of holistic healers, it was all about removing toxins, cleansing the gut and liver first, then replenishing with nutrient-dense, whole foods that provided all the building blocks to produce healthy cells.

It worked. After three months, my cell values were still bad, but I was feeling so much better that I chose to continue eating raw food. After nine months, my cell values were getting better, and after one year, I was cancer free. Today, I am a mom of three beautiful, healthy, and smart sons.

At first, I resisted the change from eating everything to eating raw plants only! I ridiculed the message my dad was trying to tell me. I was in disbelief. If it would be so easy to heal something as dangerous as cancer, how is it that scientists were still spending hundreds of thousands of dollars on research for a cure? Today, healing the physical body and keeping it healthy with food is the most natural thing to me. How could I ever not know that? I learned to listen to my body's needs and that food is energy. I call this the **Miracle of Becoming.**

During that same year, I was training with friends on a new trampoline. I felt fear of jumping somersaults but tried to force myself to do it anyway. There was a conflict between trying to commit and not letting go of fear. Of course, I learned that the hard way when I failed to estimate the jumping height correctly and fractured three vertebrae.

Again, everyone said the falling height wasn't high enough to cause fractures in a young person like myself. Again, the doctors ordered surgery and planned to put in a titanium rod, stiffening five vertebrae. Again, it didn't make sense to me. When every other bone in the body can heal naturally, why shouldn't vertebrae be able to? I didn't want to take chances with titanium screws. After I refused this procedure, another doctor suggested injecting a surgical concrete mixture into the vertebrae. My answer was no. I would not agree to a treatment that would block nutrients from getting where they were needed for healing.

The spinal nerves of the vertebrae I broke connect to the uterus and ovaries. Their fragility had nothing to do with the physical body or the density of my bones. It had everything to do with self-respect and living feminine flow on the energetical level.

I chose to let my spine heal conventionally. It took two months before I could get out of bed and into a wheelchair, attempting to use a real restroom again. During the weeks of laying in a hospital bed, I had friends visit me every day. They brought me fresh fruits and salads, and the ones who couldn't visit called and read books to me on the phone. Their loving support gave me the courage to be patient! Yoga and breathwork became part of my daily routine, already while still laying in a hospital bed not being able to sit up.

Yoga rebuilt the inner core to support the spine, while breathwork fine-tuned my awareness of the energy channels. Only one year later, I moved to Shanghai to start doctoral research on urban planning, moving just fine again. The awareness of being more than a physical body, consciously noticing the subtler qualities is what I call the **Miracle of Befriending the Energy Body.**

Fast-forward to the year 2010.

Meanwhile, my husband and I were living in the United States as we moved there for work. I had a teaching assignment at a lovely Jesuit college. We got married so that we could make this big move as a family. The boys were still so little and couldn't even speak English yet. Then, our marriage began to crumble. It was fast and brutal. Our fights occurred more frequently, turning ugly and violent. It came to the point that the children and I flew home to my mom, while begging him to consider counseling for us. His response came two weeks later by mail: he had filed a criminal lawsuit against me citing the Hague Convention for Child Abduction, requesting the court to put me to jail as a kidnapper, sending our boys who were all born in Germany to him.

Luckily, the judge didn't go for it, but I was ordered to return to the US as our place of permanent residence to complete our divorce. I was so naïve and didn't know anything about family law or trial proceedings, nor was I prepared for the timeline ahead. Upon my return, there was more mail waiting. It was a court order stating the children and I were not allowed to leave the country as long as the divorce was pending with regard to the recent kidnapping case. I tried to go back to teaching at the college, but he had alerted them that we were going through divorce; thus, my work visa was about to expire soon.

It didn't take long for me to run out of money. My sons and I ended up being homeless. I forced myself to smile at the children during the day but at night I was consumed by despair. I asked my lawyer, how I was supposed to feed my children? I could not work legally anymore, was not allowed to go home, and did not receive child support due to the pending divorce. He said, "You cannot work anymore, but you can always employ yourself." I started digging in my brain for a skill that I could turn into a source of revenue, fast.

German bread! I knew how to bake! At first, friends let me use their kitchen and I took hearty sourdough breads to the local farmer's market. They were a huge success. After a short while, I was able to negotiate a commercial lease and established Manna Bakery LLC, our town's first organic bakery. The business grew quickly. I purchased equipment at auctions and started supplying local coffee shops and restaurants, yet I was stressed-out beyond words, fearing that at any point in time someone could find out that my visa was about to expire. I was stuck in a legal dilemma between immigration and family law, and once again, had to find a solution fast. My lawyer warned me saying, "Manja, if you had to leave this country, you would be forced to leave the children here and there would be no way that you would ever get custody again because the court would interpret it as abandonment."

How was this possible? How could it be legal that I had never done anything but taking care of my children, and now I found myself having to prove that I'm a good mother and not a criminal? Meanwhile, my ex-husband found ever-new excuses to postpone the trial and I found myself drowning in depression and debt, making it hard to get up and keep pushing every day. Some days, the despair grew so intense that I thought I could not bear this suffering any longer. For months in a row, I woke up in the morning and my only thought was, "You need to stay alive, Manja, the boys need you." And every evening, I would sigh, *I survived another day.* It was an awfully draining struggle.

One night, the boys were in bed, I broke down in tears and poured myself a glass of cheap wine. Suddenly, my oldest son came back out of his room, put a CD into his player and said, "Mommy, I think you really need to hear this", and he went back to his bed. Out of the speakers came an old U2 song, "You've got to get yourself together, you are stuck in a moment, and now you can't get out of it ..." Bang! Did I just receive a wake-up slap from my six-year-old? That very moment, I realized that I had allowed negative circumstances and sad feelings to do even more bad stuff to myself. I poured the wine down the drain and started meditating every night. Going into deep Chöd-trances, one by one, I transformed my shadows into allies and put myself back together.

And then I had an aha-moment: I owned an LLC! Manna Bakery could file for an employer-sponsored work visa for me. Easier said than done; in order to qualify as a sponsor, Manna Bakery was required to create jobs for Americans. So, I hired three women as bakers and one part-time janitor and submitted the visa application. Their wages and the legal fees ate up all my profit but, again, I was a mom and would never allow my children to be separated from me. I was working 80+ hours per week, bringing the boys to the kitchen after school, feeding them there, baking while they would do homework, and even putting them to sleep at the kitchen. My boys and I were living on a budget of $12,000 per year. I was terrified that someone could say, "She cannot provide well enough for the children."

Finally, we went to trial and I was awarded full custody. This was the biggest win I could have hoped for as it gave me my children and my freedom back.

At first, after putting in so much effort, I thought I would build the bakery into a bigger business. But after four and a half years, I was exhausted to the bones, so I sold everything. One thing from the trial that was particularly stuck in my head was how the judge said, "Why would she need child support? She has a PhD and he is only an engineer. If she wanted to, she could make ten times as much money." She said it with such remarkable casualness. There was no cynicism or doubt behind these words, but she meant it. I wondered what she saw that I didn't. It dawned on me that I had adopted an identity of being poor, intimidated, and feeling like I was swimming against the current. What nonsense!

I still felt clueless about living life successfully, but I had learned that in order for things to change, we need to be ready to abandon our stories about them. Sometimes, we need to take a detour in our lives—like I did with my bakery—but that doesn't change our purpose. What we believe to know is never complete. Knowledge evolves as our needs evolve. At the time, I felt like I couldn't see the forest because there were too many trees in the way. I learned that my thoughts can lie to me and do not define who I am.

It was high time to do something to get a better overview. I saved some money and booked a flight lesson, and before I knew it, I found myself sitting in a small Cessna next to a handsome flight instructor, holding the yoke in my hands and flying over white sand beaches down the Gulf Coast. What an eye opener! Life is so beautiful, abundant, and comes with a wide-open horizon! I learned that we can change the meaning that we assign to our stories and that we can choose to end relationships we have with painful stories. I learned that thoughts are energy. I call this the **Miracle of Insight.**

Fast-forward to the year 2020.

I am still cancer free, and my spine is flexible and pain-free. The boys are grown into healthy and smart young men. I love my husband, home, and am blessed to do work that brings me joy. We love to travel a lot as a family, and I host yoga and energy healing retreats. For the most recent yoga and energy healing retreats, I took groups to visit the Mayan jungle in Belize, the hot springs in Rincon de la Vieje, Costa Rica, the ancient Greek temples in Sicily, and the beaches in Destin, Florida. Oh, delicious freedom!

This is the secret of resilience and of realizing our full potential: alignment with purpose. It works like connecting conduits in an electrical circuit; everything comes into a flow. The best part is that when we act with purpose, we are naturally good at it. Life gets easier and prosperity is created abundantly.

As human beings, we don't have energy, we generate it. We have to ignite our inner power with purpose so exciting and fulfilling that our thoughts transcend any perceived imperfections and our consciousness expands in every direction. We also share this generously with others so that dormant talents become alive and we discover creative solutions for ourselves and one another whenever needed. It is overcoming our separateness, celebrating blessings with others, and shifting from ego-mode into consciousness-mode. I call this the **Miracle of Unbecoming.**

About the Author

Dr. Manja H. Podratz, PhD

Manja was born and raised in East Germany. She holds a PhD in Theory of Architecture and in Media Studies, a BA in Arts Management and Cultural Studies, and a BA in Integrative Medicine. She taught college level for 11 years in Germany, Italy, and the United States, and contributed to several academic books and articles published both in English and German during this time. Currently, she is a PhD student with Quantum University.

Manja lives with her husband and sons in Mobile, Alabama, where she offers energy healing, brain health coaching, hypnotherapy, and acupuncture, as well as teaching yoga and meditation. She helps her clients to heal trauma, overcome limiting beliefs, and remember what brings them joy. Frequently, she teaches group programs on diet and hormonal balance, cancer prevention, healing from Lyme disease, and how to bridge the communication gap with autistic persons. Her favorite thing to do is hosting international yoga and energy healing retreats.

She is the author of *Das Leben kennt den Weg* (2006), a guidebook about natural pregnancy and childbirth as well as vegan nutrition during pregnancy, currently being updated and translated into English, and *Von mir aus... Bewegter Leib – Fluechtiger Raum* (2008), a study about the architectural movement space.

Her motto in life is:

"If you've been given much, it is your responsibility to give much back and serve your family and your community for the highest good of all."

Contact Information:

Websites:
www.drmanjapodratz.com
www.yogawithmanja.com
Email: manja@drmanjapodratz.com
Telephone: 1 (251) 234-4771

HEALING THROUGH A
BROKEN HEART

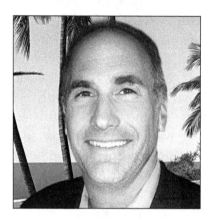

Dr. Jeffrey Benton

I am and have been a nerve system rehabilitation specialist specializing in trauma neutralization for over 20 years. My doctoral training occurred at the Southern California University of Health Sciences where I earned my Doctor of Chiropractic in 1996. Over the years I have added numerous certifications. My awakening and subsequent miracle story started early in my career in the health sciences.

I'm a first generation holocaust survivor's child. I am the middle child of parents who miraculously lived through the Holocaust (1938–1945). During that time, my parents, who had not yet met each other, separately witnessed and experienced unimaginable depravity of life. They saw systematic murder, desecration of human values, and total lack of respect for the human spirit.

It is difficult for us to fathom the enormous degree to which living through this traumatic experience impacted their lives.

Witnessing horrific, catastrophic atrocities could never be forgotten, no matter how deeply they pushed them into their subconscious.

My parents' overwhelming fear of the unknown (not knowing if they were going to live or die during the holocaust) permeated our home with "anxious energy," making it difficult for me to stay focused. The psycho-emotional impact of what they endured was transferred to the family by invisible threads of unease.

My siblings and I were bathed in this nervous family atmosphere. My parents provided us with the basics, a bed to sleep in and food to eat. We were not a cuddly, physically affectionate family. I did not receive tools such as empathy and physical touching that would have developed a healthier sense of self-esteem, which we mistook for normal.

In my youth, I was always curious about life and was forever seeking to understand the human body. I was intrigued and fascinated by the human body and loved fixing things. In retrospect it seems that it was natural for me to have put these two passions together. Both are about how I can make body and spirit better and help them function with poise. Following my instincts, and angelic guidance, I moved towards a career in healing and became a licensed chiropractor.

My Heart Broken Open

In my 30s, I dated a very special woman whom I believed to be a soulmate. Early in my chiropractic career I came to work in a chiropractic office where I met an acupuncturist. We began working together, which led to dating. She felt the magical connection between us almost immediately. In contrast I was blind to the reality of how deep and spiritual our connection really was. It was only after we had broken up that I realized what I had lost.

I did not appreciate how special and rare this feeling is until it was too late. The lady in question, however, did understand the rarity of what we had and waited for me to feel it as well. We even went to a therapist to discuss our relationship. I broke up with her at the conclusion of that session. This was devastating news for her and, walking away from that session, we agreed that we should end our relationship.

Literally 24 hours later, I awoke with a devastating feeling—I was struck down with a mighty blow. Something really heavy had crushed my spirit. It was an unrelenting crushing pain of despair. I realized it was the loss of her love. I fully understood the words of Bette Middler's song "Wind beneath my Wings," because the wind was gone, and I was falling. I called her crying, sobbing uncontrollably, that I was wrong and let her know how much I love her and miss her. But from her point of view, this was 24 hours too late. I had woken up from my immature ambivalence 24 hours too late. She told me that she had been seeing someone else as friends and had accepted his invitation to date after our therapy session.

My heartbreak was a catalyst to several personal awakenings. I realized that I truly loved her, and this forced me to deal with my invisible strings of anxiety, my broken heart, and many other issues. My meltdown was so tumultuous; I could have ended up at a psychiatric ward or worse had I not taken classes, attended prayer connections, and made use of the spiritual tools offered at the Kabbalah Centre in Los Angeles. There, I learned many empowering skills to raise my consciousness and transform my life through intention, prayer, and meditation.

As I cried to God for help, I distinctly heard a voice in my head asking me was I sure I wanted her back. Without hesitation I answered, "Yes! One hundred percent!" I had ingested the red pill. My journey to discover what I needed to accomplish in order to get the love of my life back had begun. My ex-girlfriend at this time told me to do the work I needed to do at the Kabbalah Centre. She really didn't want to see me and put me on this path. Little did she know that I would really listen to her. Using the sacred teachings and sanctification process I felt like I ascended into the heavens without a balloon.

This roller coaster of an experience in the upper levels of consciousness is indescribable. I felt like I was floating in the ether somewhere between Yesod and Tiphareth for weeks on end. My bills weren't paid, I could hardly keep things together I was so ungrounded. I can really understand why the study of Kabbalistic thought should be relegated to someone who is well grounded, of which I was not. This entire journey of surreal proportions occurred entirely without mind-altering drugs or medication.

Something huge was happening to my body and mind. I noticed that I was losing weight and vividly remember feeling so starved that I voraciously pulled out three rib steaks out of the freezer, broiling them just enough and scarfing them down like my brain was starving, literally starving for protein. Something had unlocked within me.

Another time, I be friended several like-minded spiritual sojourners. One night, at the conclusion of a meeting, one of the other participants, a reiki teacher, offered to give me a session, which I accepted. As I sat straight in a chair and her hands were moving around my head, I started to feel sparks emanating from my head, and my hair smelled like it was on fire! I was too clear of a vessel, and the energy that this loving practitioner wanted to share with me was too much.

This time of my life was especially painful on my heart and my soul. Several weeks after this episode, I had fallen asleep in my futon couch at my apartment to the songs of ABBA, only to awaken at 5:00 a.m. with tears gushing down my face and my heart painfully on fire. It felt as if rusted iron leaves covering up my heart were pushed open, exposing the vulnerable heart chakra beneath. It was an out-of-this-world sensation.

A minute later, at 5:01, the phone rang. I picked it up and heard her sobbing. She was crying just as painfully and hard as I was. We expressed our heartfelt love for each other and the synchronous agony we both felt, which was only for each other. We were on the phone for an hour, crying and sobbing, expressing our mutual love.

Angelic Help

One afternoon, I was at my apartment, and heard hundreds of voices (which I believe to be angels) screaming into my head, telling me that she was engaged. I freaked out. I ran downstairs not knowing what to do. I looked down, and in the gutter, I saw three rings: a butterfly ring and two others. I knew that this was a sign that I needed to do something. If I wanted her, I needed to propose marriage to her and her two children—hence the three rings. I grabbed the rings, cleaned them up, drove over to her home and told her that she could not marry this other person; that I loved her, and I wanted to marry her. I gave her the butterfly ring. She was in shock, not just because I had proposed to her, but because how could I know? The other man had just proposed to her earlier that day! All of a sudden, she had two proposals. Needless to say she was at her own crossroads. SShe eventually chose not to accept either proposal, deciding rather to focus on her children for the time being.

When I cried out to God, not only did I beseech God for tools to help me heal my aching heart and soul, I also asked for tools to help my soul mate heal her emotional wounds. I knew that I had to rebuild trust with her and her children to even have the possibility of re-establishing the magical connection that was broken between us.

This was no small task. During this period of healing and self-discovery, I realized my cultural view at that time was that I desired to find a single woman with no baggage (which I interpreted as someone who does not have children). This wonderful woman had two children, whom I subconsciously labeled as not desirable, instead of embracing an opportunity to be part of their lives. I was not big enough to accept the particular challenges to embrace a wonderful woman with children. As I look back, I recognize that I had been asleep and ignorant of this beautiful light in my life, which I lost. By the time I awoke from my obliviousness, it was too late.

The Emotional Trauma Release Technique™ was born during this time of deep, deep inner growth and self-evolution. When used individually, this technique is designed to help you heal your inner child from the hurt and the pains of early life. When used in a relationship, it helps unblock and unleash the energy blocks that keep people apart.

We met up several weeks after I presented her with the butterfly engagement ring. We went for a little walk holding each other's hands. It felt to me like we were not walking on the ground but instead floating on air. We did not say a word to each other and were just present together, experiencing this bliss.

She eventually broke up with the other person she was dating. We got back together and began working together again. I felt that I had grown since we had first broken up but obviously there was still more to do. I believe she saw that I did the work that merited me to be with her again. That is when the real work of the relationship needed to begin.

There is a well-known saying: "Physician, heal thyself." This experience forced me to look at myself and examine who I was. I continued taking classes at the Kabbalah Centre, combined with the many healing modalities that I had studied at Chiropractic College, helped me elevate my consciousness to a higher vibration. I was finally able to stand still in a relaxed pose. I no longer felt that anxious energy, which had impacted my childhood. The symbiotic relationship between hurtful heartbreak and healing became apparent. After much time and effort, the Emotional Trauma Release Technique was born.

The Birth of the Emotional Trauma Release Technique™

A young lady was referred to the Light Touch Healing Center for pain and tight muscles. She had been in psychiatric care for ten days at Cedars Sinai Hospital. The person referring this young lady to us explained that she was admitted because it seemed that she had deliberately driven into the yellow barrels filled with water that buttress the freeway off ramp.

I sat down with her and explained the muscle testing process. This is also known as Applied Kinesiology testing and this process assesses the neurological integrity of different body parts by assessing muscle strength. After checking her neck and upper body, I turned my attention to her legs. She held her left arm out in front of her, as I applied downward pressure. Her left arm went weak when I touched her right thigh, indicating something was wrong. I did not see any visible markings on her skin, like a scar or a discoloration. I asked her if anything had happened to this area of her body. Her demeanor changed as she told me that she had been sexually assaulted while on a date. "That's where he grabbed me," she said. The assailant, a date, grabbed her by the thigh and pulled her down.

I was secretly freaking out. I never had this kind of experience come up in the past. I stayed calm and proceeded to have her breathe while thinking about the event. I gently extended her head back an inch on the inhale and back to neutral on the exhale. This simple process helped ease the anxiety and traumatic memory of that event. The rest of the visit was focused on clearing all the different places that date rape trauma effected—her self-esteem, her heart, her trust in herself, her trust in men, to name a few.

This single visit took about two hours, and it was one that shifted her life. She experienced relief from the physical ills and explained that she also felt the release and removal of the emotional trauma and resultant blockages that had been driving her to distraction. She now could think clearly and felt a return of her power. No longer did she let that adverse event define her. She could return to her productive and positive life. Clearing this trauma allowed her to trust herself and to trust men again. She returned to school and was able to find the man of her dreams. A year later, she invited me to her wedding!

At the time, I didn't know what I had done. It turns out that this was the first time the Emotional Trauma Release Technique™ was used. This patient wrote me a long letter.

Here is an excerpt:

> I felt so much energy radiating from Dr. Benton. I felt weak and dizzy for a second but a few minutes later my heart was filled with comforting warmth and joy. He talked to me and explained it to me slowly all the barriers that I have to overcome. Most of my barriers had to do with spiritual world. There was a curse put on me six years ago in Dr. Benton had help to clear out of my system from the remaining of that curse. He cleared my aura and my spirits vibrated from the lights that we send it on me at the third eye. We both share the same idea about "Color Therapy Healing" and the techniques that are still to be developed and yet to come.
>
> Last but not least, he didn't ask me for any rewards or payments, he helped me from the bottom of his heart. He worked on me for two hours and we spent quite a bit of time talking. I formed friendship ties with Benton's family

including mother who gave me a warm greeting. Kindness makes the world go round. One trip to Dr. Benton's office saved me years of therapy to come, more medication to fill my blood flow and more support group time. I was cleared spiritually and physically and the most important thing I stopped overeating and feeling depressed. I am looking forward into helping Dr. Benton in every way I can.

This story reflects how the power of a heart broken open, and trust in God can heal the world of past hurt. From this extremely painful and transformative spiritual journey, the Emotional Trauma Release Technique™ was born. This technique has since been used to help countless people shift their lives from victimhood to creator. The Emotional Trauma Release Technique™ allows you to get out of the rut life put you in.

You can find out more about this technique in the book, Emotional Trauma Release Technique: The Ultimate System for Releasing Life Traumas, due out Summer 2020.

You can find videos and more information at www.etrt.org.

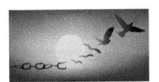

The Emotional Trauma Release Technique™ unchains you from your past and lets you fly into your future.

About the Author

Dr. Jeffrey Benton, DC, CTN, ACN, QME

Jeffrey is a licensed chiropractic and naturopathic healer who has spent his life studying and optimizing the entire human being. This includes the physical body, the mind, and the spirit. In addition to using advanced physical therapy modalities, he uses humor and appreciation to switch on the body's internal self-correcting programs to improve the human potential.

He received his Bachelor of Science in Biology in 1990 from California State University, Northridge, and his Doctor of Chiropractic in 1996 from Southern California University of Health Sciences. He has special training in the advanced techniques including Chiropractic Kinesiology, Zindler C.M.R.T. acupressure, and Cranial Adjusting Turner Style. He is certified in

Applied Clinical Nutrition and a Qualified Medical Examiner for the State of California. He has received numerous certifications in advanced studies in nutrition and the biomechanics of low-impact injuries. These techniques, coupled with massage and proven sports rehabilitation therapies, maximize your body's physical magnificence and effectiveness.

He was selected as a Top Chiropractor by *Los Angeles Magazine* for the past three years and received the Health Professional of the Year award in 2019 from Eric Zuley and EZWay TV.

He is recognized for his understanding that as we go through life, trauma and traumatic events rarely heal completely and often leaves remnants that slows the body down and causes aging.

As part of his post-doctorate studies, Dr. Benton has developed the Emotional Trauma Release Technique™. This advanced technology uses kinesiology and nurturing attention to help neutralize the anxiety of past events. Results are often immediate and astounding.

He has lectured at the Academy of Integrative Health and Medicine, the Brentwood Chamber of Commerce, USC Pain Medicine Clinic, Academy of Complimentary Integrative Medicine, Biogenesis Summit, and numerous other organizations.

Contact Information:

Website: www.lighttouchhealingcenter.com
Telephone: (323) 297-0566
Facebook: Jeffrey D. Benton
Instagram: LTHCenter
LinkedIn: drjeffreybenton

MIRACULOUS RESULTS WITH MAGNA WAVE PEMF

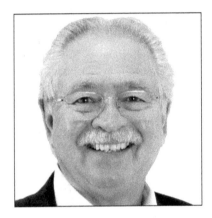

Pat Ziemer

Miracle: An event so marvelous that it seems like it is from above.

Miracle is a noun meaning an amazing or wonderful occurrence.

As a business owner and product developer, I have always been told not to say that a product is a miracle or that there is a secret to how something works because people are often skeptical of such statements. However, over the years, I have come to expect amazing or wonderful occurrences with the use of our machines. Many of our practitioners and customers have called their results "Magna Wave Machine Miracles." I often say, "Don't believe in miracles, work toward them and depend on them."

In this chapter, I will provide you with an overview of PEMF and how Magna Wave PEMF utilizes this therapy for human health and wellness. There are two types of PEMF equipment: low voltage, low frequency, and high voltage, low frequency. The difference between the two is the speed of results. Low voltage PEMF is sufficient but slower to achieve results, while high voltage PEMF often provides faster and sometimes, instantaneous results. Magna Wave PEMF devices are high voltage, low-frequency devices.

Inflammation is the number one cause of pain in the body. The use of Pulsed Electromagnetic Fields (PEMF) provides a means to reduce inflammation, thereby reducing and relieving pain. The primary function is to improve oxygenation and improve blood flow in the body. Magnetic fields affect the charge of the cell membrane, which opens up the cell membrane channels. These channels are like the doors and windows of a house for airflow and circulation. By opening cell channels, nutrients are easily absorbed by the cell and waste easily eliminated. The process helps to rebalance and restore optimum cell function. If you utilize PEMF to restore cells continually, they will all work more efficiently. By using PEMF for restoring or maintaining cellular function, you will in turn repair or maintain organ function, allowing the entire body to function better and maintain wellness. The method provides for the body to be in a position to heal itself better and to better utilize medications provided for the healing process.

A new angle on Alzheimer's, depression, anxiety, strokes, and concussions is the inflammation connection. Recent studies have shown how the immune system and inflammation play a role in the development of these indications. Targeting specific elements of the inflammatory process could be useful in treating or preventing these and other disorders. Various drugs and medications are given to fight the body's inflammation processes.

The use of Magna Wave PEMF has demonstrated the promise of a drug-free method of fighting the damaging effects of inflammation as a part of the disease. The PEMF modality has gained FDA clearance for uses that include; non-union fractures, depression, autism, incontinence, and brain tumors. The PEMF modality is used regularly to improve any indication that could benefit from improved oxygenation and inflammation reduction. The list of positive result uses is long and growing, including everything from arthritis to stress-related diseases and speedier recovery.

Future Brain Health Machine Miracles

The incidence of concussions and traumatic brain injuries (TBI) represents a rising concern in the area of sports, military activities, and work injuries. As reported in the Journal of Neurology (Brain 2019:142255-262), there is a scientifically proven method for measuring brain voltage using a combination of a quantitative electroencephalogram (QEEG) coupled with a test known as the P300 (Evoked Potential). The available research shows that brain voltage typically drops following a concussion and is the last physiological measurement to return to a healthy state following a head injury.

Quite often, the only medical advice given to the post-concussion patient is to rest. However, there might be other mechanisms by which an individual can recover more efficiently while reducing the risk of future concussions. Magna Wave is currently working with Dr. Larry Lyons, a psychologist in San Diego, California in researching the use of high-powered PEMF to increase brain voltage and improve brainpower or neural output. The brain and body will mimic the PEMF fed into it, and capillary blood flow will increase. Inflammation can limit the success of other types of biofeedback; PEMF can reduce inflammation while administered at fast speeds without generating heat and damaging tissue. PEMF can be used to entrain the brain via operant conditioning or disentrain the brain via dishabituation. It is hypothesized that in the brain, PEMF increases nitric oxide, which induces vasodilation, enhances microvascular perfusion and tissue oxygenation, and may be a useful adjunct therapy in traumatic brain injury.

In the present San Diego study, participants undergo a quantitative electroencephalogram (QEEG) to obtain a baseline measure of their brain voltage. The participants then receive a total of six PEMF sessions over three weeks using the Magna Wave system. For treatment, the coils are placed on the temporal regions of the brain. The participants are then retested with the quantitative electroencephalogram (QEEG) to determine brain voltage (i.e., how many neurons fire in unison when a novel stimuli is presented in the P300 auditory task) and brain speed (how fast does it take for the brain to recognize a change in stimuli) changes.

By examining brain speed with brain voltage, an approximate brain age can be calculated. By breaking down the test results down to the phrase "brain age," it becomes an easy reference point for a person to comprehend. It will be interesting to see if high-powered PEMF as administered by the Magna Wave technology can create a more youthful brain. The formula presented is: BRAIN SPEED (in milliseconds) X BRAIN POWER (voltage) = BRAIN AGE.

While the study is ongoing, patients are running through the study with very good preliminary results. One pre-post WAVI (QEEG) result in this study; we have a 56-year-old woman with chronic back pain. She has had a total of eight PEMF sessions in over ten weeks. Here are the results:

3/13/2019 EEG Brain Speed: 284 milliseconds, EEG Brain Power: 5.0 microvolts

1/24/2020 EEG Brain Speed: 240 milliseconds, EEG Brain Power: 10.0 microvolts

Her brain processing speed increased by 15%, and her brainpower increased by 103%. These are fantastic results. Also, the Magna Wave PEMF pulsed treatment helped her stop all prescribed pain medications. I see this as a great beginning to what many could see as miraculous results in brain health with Magna Wave PEMF therapy.

My Wife Debi and the Miracle Machine

Debi was a schoolteacher, and she had taken a fall on ice while walking her students between buildings in 2005. As a result, she had severe compression of her upper spine, and she had three herniated discs. She experienced continual pain and limited mobility of her left arm and shoulder. I used all of the devices available to us, including low power PEMF and laser therapy, to try to help her situation. While she gained some relief, she did not experience any reversal of the case.

In 2007, a horse trainer friend of mine at the Santa Anita racetrack in California called me and told me about this high-powered PEMF machine they were using on their horses and how well it was working. That same day while at a horse show in Atlanta, a customer came up to me and told me about a similar device. I felt that someone was trying to tell me something, so I called the manufacturers. It turns out that both were going to be at an anti-aging conference in Orlando, Florida. We decided to go and find out firsthand about this high-powered PEMF product.

While attending a machine demonstration session at the show, they asked for a volunteer from the audience to try the machine. Debi looked at me and said that she would do it because nothing had worked for her and that this new machine probably would not work either, then we could leave and go back to Ocala. She volunteered, went to the stage, sat in a chair, and had her shoulder treated for eight minutes. When she stood up and went to move her arm as directed, she had complete mobility and no pain in her back or shoulder. With tears in her eyes, as she looked at me, and I immediately knew that we were going to have to find a way to get this miracle machine.

We worked a deal with one of the manufacturers and bought a machine and began a continuous treatment regimen that gave her total mobility and no pain. For the past 15 years, her protocol has been two to three 20-minute treatments, which gives her three to four weeks of no pain and complete mobility. Her doctors still question why she has no pain or mobility issues when they look at her X-rays.

Another Debi Machine Miracle

In 2004, Debi was diagnosed with an ascending aortic aneurysm at just under three centimeters in size, with five centimeters considered as very serious. It became routine that she would return to the doctor every six months for an MRI to monitor the situation to ensure that it was not getting any larger. At the time, she was treating our boxer's hip dysplasia with a low-power device to avoid the dog needing surgery hopefully.

She would lay in a coil with the dog during the treatments. The machine miracle is that the dog never required surgery and when Debi returned to her doctor for her next MRI for her aneurysm, the results showed that it had reduced in size, to which the doctor said seemed impossible because aneurysms don't shrink. She continued to treat the dog periodically and thus herself over the next couple of years with little change to the aneurysm. As previously mentioned, in 2007 we began using the high-powered PEMF devices and she continued her treatment regimen. At the time we were traveling full time in our RV bus promoting and building our business.

Consequently in 2008 and 2009, she missed her biannual check-ups for her aneurysm. When we stopped traveling full-time in 2010 and returned to Louisville, she scheduled an appointment to see her doctor. He gave her a stern lecture for not keeping up with her check-ups and then scheduled an MRI. When the results came back, he called her to the office and informed her that the aneurysm was gone. He explained that it must have been a misdiagnosis from the beginning because he could not figure out what had happened and of course, he would not discuss or consider the potential effects of PEMF. With four years of supporting MRIs, he did not know what to say because this does not happen to diagnosed aneurysms. To us, this was clearly a Magna Wave machine miracle.

Parkinson's Machine Miracle

Karen bought her Magna Wave machine to treat her horses and her husband Harry, who suffers from Parkinson's disease. He had been diagnosed two or three years before her getting her machine. It was a fast progressing kind, and it looked like he had already had it for 10 years; he had lost 75% of function of the left side of his body and was stumbling and dragging his foot. He could not grab anything with his left hand. He could not work with tools, which left him depressed because his hobby and his gift from God is building beautiful furniture. Harry stopped building and he became angry and cranky because he knew he was losing his life and everything he enjoyed.

With the first treatment, nothing much happened. Second treatment, still nothing. After the third treatment, Harry said, "Wow, I really feel better. I feel really good." That night, he did not have to take his pain medicine or his sleeping medicine to go to bed. So after the third treatment, we had already stopped two of his 10 medications that he was on, and with each treatment he has just gotten better and better.

So after six months of treatments, Harry began building furniture again. He returned to work and is building a $14 million wastewater treatment plant in Texas. You have to be 100% mentally alert for being responsible for this kind of work, and with Parkinson's, it affects the entire body physically, mentally, and emotionally. The machine has helped reverse his disease symptoms and more than 50% of the physical damage. It has also helped him mentally and emotionally and has improved the metabolization of his medications, which helps them to work better. In the three and a half years that she treated him, his medicine has not been increased or even changed, and if you know anything about Parkinson's, you have to change it every six months to a year to intensify it, or you have to change the medication completely. In the last report, Harry has decreased his number of prescriptions from 10 to five and continues to see improvement.

I am continually amazed at the results people receive with the utilization of this PEMF miracle machine. Health and wellness utilizing Magna Wave PEMF is my passion. My daughter Alane Paulley now runs the day-to-day operations of the company, which allows me to now dedicate my life and time to helping thousands of people to gain health, wellness, and the success in their life that they desire. I thank God every day for the opportunity to do this. I am available to help; just let me know.

* These devices are not meant to heal or cure any condition or disease and or not yet approved by the FDA. They are intended for energy supplementation, always contact your physician before beginning new supplements or procedures.

About the Author

Pat Ziemer

Pat is the owner of Magna Wave. He has been working full time with PEMF since 2002. The company's therapy devices are used extensively on racehorses, performance horses, and professional athletes. Seven recent Kentucky Derby winners and numerous world champions in many horse disciplines utilize the therapy regularly. In 2007, Pat acquired the rights to the PEMF device, repackaged it, branded it as Magna Wave and hit the road marketing the Magna Wave brand. Since 2007 the company has placed over 3000 Magna Wave devices into the market for private and professional use. Magna Wave now services the human, small animal, and equine markets.

Contact Information:

For additional information and additional miracle machine, testimonials visit: MagnaWavePEMF.com or contact Pat directly at PatZiemer@ MagnaWavePEMF.com. You can find him on LinkedIn under the name of Patrick Ziemer.

A JOURNEY INTO MIRACLES

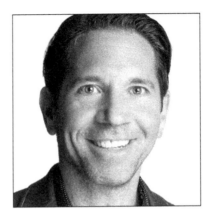

Dr. Jared Leon

Imagine a life filled with happiness, love, great friends, and family—even a wonderful, fulfilling job. Sounds too good to be true, correct? Well, that was myself four years ago when I had been a functional chiropractor working in my very blessed private practice helping many patients achieve optimal health. I had just finished changing my focus from chiropractic to functional neurology and just finished my two-year arduous journey of classwork, 200 hours of credit requirements of post-doctrine neurology and about six months of intense study for my neurology boards.

I had flown out to Atlanta from New York to go take a test that would change my life and allow me to check off a dream of receiving my diplomate in functional neurology. To my dismay, three long months of waiting for results after taking the eight-hour written test on day one and an intense practical exam on day two, I received an email that would rock me to my core. It simply said that I passed the practical part of the test but failed the written part. Reading this sent a jolt through my nervous system for many reasons but looking back now it had really been my first major failure in over two decades. So, after a quick and horrible realization of defeat and that I could not take the test again until next year, I figured I would suck it up, put on a fake smile, and go to my practice and continue helping my patients.

That night, after gently falling to sleep for about two hours, I was woken up with the most intense migraine headache of my life. The throbbing and stabbing pain into my right eye was so intense that by the time I threw myself out of bed and looked in the mirror, my eye had looked almost closed with my pupil looking extremely big and the white sclera of my eye was bloodshot with uncontrollable tears leaking out of it. It's about 1:00 in the morning and my wife and kids are sleeping and I am standing in front of the bathroom mirror thinking, "What can I do and what is wrong with me?" So, of course the unhealthy and negative thoughts start dancing in my head that I am either having a stroke or the worst migraine of my life, and that I may have to wake the family and go to the hospital. Then either by intense pride or my strong beliefs of natural healing, I decided that if I could just make it down to the couch and take some Advil (which I try to never take), I would be fine after drinking some water and by placing ice on my head and neck.

After feeling no relieve and the pain further intensifying, I decided to take some Fioricet, a migraine medication that was prescribed many years ago when I had a series of lesser bouts. At this point the probability of the medication working was lessened by how old the medication was and loss of bioavailability. Plus, it really only works well if taken right at the onset of the migraine. Sadly, the medications just slightly reduced the intensity of my pain. After experiencing some of the worst head pain of my life, it's now morning and the sun was rising, as well as my family. I must have looked pretty fatigued from the look of my wife's concerned face thereby forcing me to come clean of the night's endeavors. I forced myself into a cold shower and decided to man up and go to work because I had many patients who counted on me. The day was long and filled with fatigue and an innate feeling of having some of my life force being drained.

Going to bed that second night, I was exhausted and could not wait to get to bed and feel refreshed the next morning. But that deemed to be an illusion because ironically at 1:00 in the morning (again), my body jumped up with another intense migraine in the exact same location, with stabbing and throbbing right eye pain. Knowing what was going on, I ran to the bathroom again and took some medication and prayed that it would give me a little relief. Hopefully it would ward off another night of no sleep and intense pain. This horrific pattern lasted one full month, getting worse each night with less and less relief felt and adding more and more medications into my body. The days were getting harder and harder to sustain my energy and faking a positive appearance for my patients and family.

At the end of my work shifts I started feeling dizzy and headachy with the realization I should take my blood pressure. To my dismay and fear it read 200/110, which is crazy high for someone who sustains and prides themselves of being in good shape, healthy, and living a life of wellness. My intense, irregular, and abnormally high blood pressures would increase whenever stressed from any (and many daily) occurrences.

Scared, fatigued, panicked, and filled with anxiety I forced myself to my primary medical doctor for a checkup. He officially diagnosed me with severe migraines, high blood pressure, and anxiety. I was given many prescriptions from two blood pressure medications, two migraine medications, Lexapro for pain and anxiety, Valium to sleep, and a script for a brain scan to rule out a tumor. This moment in time struck me with a deep mortal and philosophical wound. Being a wellness doctor for well over a decade, I could not believe what he was saying. How could an emotional response have triggered this intense reaction that caused such havoc on my nervous system? How could I be feeling this way without a head trauma or any physical previous conditions?

In the meantime, my practice, also reducing, mirroring my poor energy and healing capacity. My home life was filled with mood swings, depression, and an extremely concerned wife, children, and family. I tried cutting-edge vitamin therapy, chiropractic adjustments, cold laser therapy, cryotherapy, BrainTap glasses to reduce my stress, Halo laser to stimulate my healing, and daily migraine meds to no prevail. After six total weeks of misery and constant 1:00 a.m. wake up calls with intense right orbital migraines that would spread around my head, I knew time was running out. I would have to turn to a true allopathic model and get the brain MRI and start to take all of the previously mentioned medications.

With my parent's intervention and advisement, I decided to go crawl into my brother's functional neurology office. Why I did not think of this idea sooner I cannot say. Fatigue and pain caused brain fog and forced all of my mental abilities just to make it through work and family life each day. After a thorough . functional neurological examination by Dr. Shannon Leon and his trusted associate Dr. Jason Langhough, they told me that they knew what was causing my migraines and that within a few weeks it would start to improve. They diagnosed me using eye goggles to see the true function of my brainstem and cerebellum, vestibular balance platform to determine my vestibular function, and a lot of the neurological tools that I had ironically just studied in my neurology program. These were used to create a treatment plan for three times each week to start to allow my brain to heal from a cortical spreading depression, an overworking brainstem, a fatigued cortical function, and bilateral posterior canal lithiasis or AKA crystals with my ears.

Within a couple of weeks of treatment, my first night of sleep had occurred and then was followed by another and then my blood pressure started to neutralize. My energy was returning, and my practice started to flourish again, but I still did not feel like myself. My mind was still overwhelmed with the causation of this event with one paramount question that kept playing over and over into my soul. Could this whole horrific episode have been from failing the test and the emotion of the failure that had locked in to my subconscious that had caused devastation on my nervous system? Which, looking back, I belief the answer was yes. Fast-forwarding to the next few months, I continued to eat clean, take my vitamins, continue getting gentle chiropractic adjustments, functional neurological checkups and corrections, and even started talking to an energetic healer (Dawn Elle from Liveinyourlight.com) to help and fortify my healing on my journey towards a medical miracle.

I was whole and energetic again after about three full months of intense healing. Wow, my miracle was here and felt and now I was inspired to start studying again for my neurology board exam and help many similar people who suffer from debilitating migraines. Is neurology and proper brain function really that important to your daily wellness? Can your brain and emotional state really control your life and all of your perceptions? YES, AND YES! An optimal life is all about creating balance and a never-ending drive for greatness while being fueled by perseverance and gratitude.

So now let's fast-forward another three years. I now have my diplomate in functional neurology and a fellowship in vestibular rehabilitation and a focus on patients who suffer the way I did. Now is a great time to reminisce and share a great miracle story that I have recently seen in my office.

Imagine a patient who walks through my clinic doors at the age of 67, accompanied by his wife who presents with a previous diagnosis of Meniere's disease. His history started off that he had recently retired from a stressful job after many years and wanted to enjoy the latter years with his wife. He describes his symptoms as debilitating, and they had ruined his retirement dreams. He described his symptoms as bilateral progressive hearing loss, right ear tinnitus (which is when you hear a loud high pitch sound that he explained as never going away, just worsening), and bouts of vertigo that occurred daily that would leave him praying in a chair for up to eight hours a day. He took a handful of medications daily to no prevail. I will never forget his laughable expression after I took his history, and looked him in the eyes and said, "I believe I can help you." His exact response was, "How can you say that after I have been to many specialists and they all told me that I am healthy and be thankful and just live with it?"

After my functional neurological examination, I sat down to review all of my findings with him and his wife. Again, thinking back, another funny moment occurred because of the fear of the unknown he was extremely skeptical and complained about the potential cost versus a lack of Medicare coverage. His wife looked him in the eyes and said, "Stop being cheap. We saved for years for the future, which you are not living well at all." In that moment our wellness journey started; I diagnosed him with a bilateral vestibular impairment and explained how treatments would entail numerous vestibular repositioning maneuvers to reduce his canal lithiasis (inner ear crystals in vestibular canals). His treatment protocol was twice a week for one month and then I would reevaluate.

With his skepticism and potential suppressed optimism, we started the process, by the end of the first week his daily eight hours of horrible chair prison reduced by half. By the end of the first month his energy was starting to return as well as his hope of a possible happy future of the retirement he once envisioned. He was now experiencing minor bouts of vertiginous symptoms with minimal downtime. Within two months of treatments he was now having days throughout the week of NO vertigo and dizziness and NO chair time; while graduating to being seen once a week. On month three, his miracle was achieved: no dizziness and vertigo at all and he was feeling better than when he was years younger. His mind regained its sharpness, his energy was improved, his vigor of life had returned, and a positive man stood before me. We hugged it out and he thanked me for all the help and regaining his life back. I reminded him of where he started and how proud I was of his commitment to heal and regain his life. In that moment, all of my arduous studies and challenges were worth it and paid back in dividends with his hug and positive experiential miracle.

As in my past pragmatic experiences, a brain not functioning optimally can have deleterious effects on quality of life. Your body is filled with an amazing innate power to heal and produce whatever it needs to create outstanding miracles from within. So, how is this forgotten so easily? Why do we always seem to surrender to fear, doubt, and worry? Why do we forget about the amazing healing capabilities of the body and seek council in a bottle, potion, or lotion? We all have an amazing and super powerful brain that we need to nurture and allow to grow continually so that we can count on it to perform miracles on a daily basis. In this state, you optimize your environment (our body) to harmonize and combat diseases, ailments, and afflictions. When our brain is out of tune and not functioning optimally, we set up an unhealthy ecosystem that is more prone to pains, diseases, and health challenges.

In conclusion, when faced with your own health challenge or crisis please remember my miracle success formula: dream or desire the outcome of what you are trying to achieve with a clear vision, followed by persistent and consistent action steps with the right amount of perseverance with a positive mindset, and watch your miracle unfold.

**Dreams + Persistent Action Steps +
Perseverance + Positive Mindset =**

Watch your Miracle Unfold

Yours in Health,
Jared A. Leon D.C., C.C.E.P., F.I.C.P.A, F.A.B.V.R., D.A.C.N.B

About the Author

Dr. Jared A. Leon, DC

Jared has embraced his work with a passion rarely seen in the healthcare community. Rather than focusing on a patient's particular symptoms, Dr. Leon concentrates upon the innate wellness harbored within the human body, thus allowing the body's natural and powerful forces to overcome afflictions.

He performs his work non-invasively, with gentle external corrections of one's own architecture to restore neural pathways from interference. Since it is ultimately these pathways that govern our health and well being, he reinforces and facilitates the neurological system's natural ability to maintain a body's health. He also utilizes high technological neurological equipment to better analyze objective information and offer cutting-edge neurological treatments and rehabilitation.

He firmly believes it is the duty of a healthcare professional to maintain wellness, by rooting out the cause of health problems, not just treating the symptoms of an illness. He strives to restore the body to peak performance, thereby minimizing the chance of illness and its debilitating results.

Contact Information:

Leon Chiropractic
213 Hallock Rd.
Suite 4B

Stony Brook, NY 11790
631-689-1000
leonchiropractic.com
drjared5@gmail.com
facebook.com/LeonChiropractic

THE TRUE NATURE OF MIRACLES

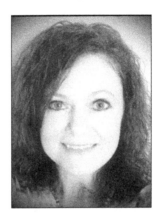

Dr. Robin J. Lambrecht

Ancient medicine isn't as mystical as it once was. Evidence presented by quantum physics has illuminated the scientific benefits of these 3,000-year-old health practices. The true nature that underlies miracles is quantum in nature. Within the energy dynamics of all substances, including the physical, there is an information flow that directs action. It is now widely known that the force that moves energy is consciousness. The energy that we don't see—our intuition, thoughts and perspectives that make up our beliefs—direct the energy and instruct our physical body.

A miracle occurs when we discover something new that shifts our beliefs, we have a new insight, the 'aha' moment where a new realization is found. In quantum physics we call this a quantum leap, where new information has changed the belief of an individual, where they now operate under the new premise.

A well-known healing concept that conventional medicine has yet been able to explain is the placebo effect. This is when a substance that has no medicinal value, such as a sugar pill, is used when conducting scientific studies to evaluate the effectiveness of a new medicine or treatment against doing nothing at all. It has been found to be as effective as the medication itself. Why? Because when we have a strong belief, and in this case, that the medicine is going to work, and trust in the practitioner providing the treatment, healing and miracles occur.

Don't underestimate the power of thoughts because they form your beliefs and direct your body processes. This is why being aware of your thoughts and transmuting them into something positive is so important. Everyone experiencing a similar situation will apply different meaning to the event based on past personal experiences and programming. The trick is trying to see as many perspectives as possible so that you have a clearer picture of what is really happening. You can create your own miracles with strong beliefs that are charged with emotions—you need both!

I have personally experienced my own healing miracles and have been witness to numerous others. But really, there is no such thing as a miracle; there is nothing random in the Universe. However, there is something even better! We can ALL create our own miracles. Why? Because the Universe is magical! It responds to you, and you can co-create with it.

This may be a little scientific for you to grasp, but it is important in understanding how your thoughts are communicated through the fabric of the Universe or matrix to create miracles. This explanation may in fact be different from your belief, but I assure you these are truths.

1. The first thing to understand is that everything in existence is a form of energy; it is just its frequency and vibration that make up how solid something is. The slower the vibration, the more solid or material it appears, so a tree's energy is slower than an animated, moving entity such as yourself and your pets.

2. The second point to consider is that everything has two sides, like a coin. The ancients refer to this as yin and yang—female and male; night and day; dark and light; cold and warm; asleep and awake. Humans are either in physical form or in energy form. We never die, we just

transition between the two sides. Therefore, there is *life after death* because energy never changes, it just moves in and out of form. So, that's good news!

An electron, is very small, has a negative charge, and moves very quickly. It is known as a particle when it is observed in some way and its second side is known as a wave. Nobel prizes have been awarded for this scientific breakthrough. So, what does this mean? An electron is responsible for ALL chemical bonds. Electrons are essential to your health because they neutralize the free radicals that damage your cells, causing inflammation that leads to numerous chronic diseases. Because of our hectic, super-stressed lifestyles and exposures to toxins, we have a very damaging positive charge. The surface of the Earth is covered with electrons, the cure that nature provides to balance our body. They move from negative to positive charge, so get outside and walk on the Earth with your bare feet. But I digress—it is the 'flip of the electron' that creates the miracle—either positive outcomes or negative, related to the direction of your thoughts and intentions. Wow, right?

3. Stress is the cause of many biochemical compound reactions that alter our state of consciousness. These are directly linked through the meaning we give to situations depending on our beliefs, the ego, and subconscious mind. In other words, you direct the electron how to act by the way you think, talk, feel and act. You instruct your body and the Universe what to do, and you have the power to alter everything that occurs in your life. That's empowerment! It is our collective thoughts, known as the noosphere, that shapes our world and the reality that we all experience. When our intentions frequency is met by another's frequency, a wave is created that makes it more powerful. So, when a group of people get together in prayer, the effect is multiplied because of the wave. Lynne McTaggart, author of *The Field*, has proven this

effect through numerous experiments. This collective consciousness is known under many different names: Higher-self, Buddha, Taoism, God, Jehovah, Chi, Prana, etc.

4. Empowerment—You are not a victim of circumstance or genes you have the power to move the energy that creates everything. Bruce Lipton explains this as epigenetics, where we change the expression of our genes in the emotional, feeling level of our body, known as the morphogenetic field. In fact, less than 1% of disease is the result of faulty genes; the rest is due to faulty thinking and the meaning we apply to things.

5. You developed most of your beliefs by the age of 7, and these beliefs created blocks in your energy system. This stagnated energy results in symptoms and then disease if it is not cleared. We have to stop living our lives on autopilot, as this is what the great awakening is all about. We now have to slow down and think before we respond, because as you know, how you deal with every thought or situation will direct either miracles or obstacles, suffering and dis-ease. We need to observe situations, be aware in the moment, and make decisions based on our authentic self, not the personality or ego self—this is where your power lies.

I have developed a course to teach you how to apply higher-order thinking with a very effective tool that allows you to enter the gap between the tic and the tock, where you have the opportunity to tap into your higher mind to create the life you deserve.

Okay, now that we know how miracles happen, let's look at a few miracles that I have witnessed and a few that I myself have lived through. I was a Registered Nurse for over 25 years, a very stressful job. I was raising four children, running an MS first dose clinic, taking my doctorate and PhD, running my own holistic health clinic, and developing a research study to help those working the front lines (paramedics, fire, police, doctors, nurses) who have developed the worst stress of all, post-traumatic stress disorder (PTSD). The study showed high clinical significance using the gold standard assessment tool the DSM-5.

Many of my clients experienced profound changes, being able to utilize the tools I use and sell, so that they become empowered to take care of their own health. Prevention is the key! Because of this, clients didn't need to continue seeing me on a regular basis unless they needed me to hold space for them, creating the wave of possibilities while they choose a new healing path. My business grew related to the referrals and the success people experienced in their lives.

- A mother of two, who works as a nurse had experienced the symptoms of PTSD for over five years. It was debilitating for her and affected her work, and especially her children. She had been to medical doctors, given anti-anxiety medication, and told she should consider quitting her job. My treatment works on the subconscious mind to affect change as well as providing her with new ways of looking at things and some tools she could use when experiencing an episode or flashback.

  It was amazing to watch the light bulb go on, appointment after appointment, the increased energy she had, the change in her thought patterns, and new meanings she applied to her past situations. The integrative approach dealing with all levels of her human experience resulted in—I dare say—a cure. The change occurred rapidly when she looked at her situation through a new perspective and changed her unconscious processing. After a month of treatments, she no longer suffered from PTSD. Four years later, she remains free of symptoms and continues to think of it as a miracle.

- One evening while working in a continuing care facility, I had a client on palliative care. He hadn't eaten in a week and was unresponsive. We had him on IV fluids and checked on him regularly to turn, apply eye drops, and ensure he was comfortable. His sister was at the bedside holding his hand. It was around 10:00 at night while I was dispensing medications that his sister came out and told me, "I think it's time." I walked to his room and checked his pulse. No pulse, no respiration. I turned off his beeping IV pump and told her I that would be right back with my stethoscope. The nursing attendant was in the room with them.

- I walked to the nursing station, took out a death certificate, grabbed my stethoscope and pen light, told the other staff that he had passed away and walked back to the room. At least three to four minutes had passed when I arrived back at the bedside. His sister was emotional, as expected in this situation, and was saying to the patient, "I wish you would have waited." Their other brother was traveling in to pay his last respects. At this time, I had the stethoscope on his chest, listening for a heartbeat. We typically listen for at least one full minute, but there was nothing. Just as I was about to take the stethoscope off his chest, I heard a beat. "It couldn't be." I must have looked a little shocked because she asked me, "What? What is it?"

- Sometimes when the body dies, there are a few responses that occur, like air leaving the chest or nerve twitches. "No, nothing." I didn't want to say anything and continued to listen. Forty seconds later, there was another beat. What was going on? His sister was rubbing his arm, crying and stating, "He's on his way. Why couldn't you just hold on a bit longer?" Then I heard another beat, he drew in a large breath in a struggle. I told her sometimes this happens as the body is shutting down. More heartbeats, then the heart started beating rapidly, over 200 beats per minute and very sporadic and irregular. This type of beat (arrhythmia) alone could cause a heart attack, so I continued to say nothing as I listened and observed in disbelief. The heartrate slowed down, and he took a struggled breath and then another one until they became more frequent. I said, "I've never seen anything like this before. His heart is now beating!" Everyone in the room was frozen in shock. His heartrate returned to normal and he was breathing more regularly. He came back from the dead! When he heard his sister pleading with him, he mustered up the strength to return for an additional two weeks, allowing his family the opportunity to say goodbye.

- I was diagnosed with polyarthritis. All of my joints were swollen, red and very painful. I couldn't walk, write, or barely move from the pain. I was put on 60 mg of Prednisone as well as narcotics. Every time they tried to taper the dose, my symptoms returned, and I was referred to a rheumatologist in Edmonton. I told him I would try to heal myself first before going to the specialist. I changed the meaning of my symptoms and believed that it was due to an acidic body. I changed the way I ate and purchased an alkaline live water machine. Very rapidly, my CRP lab level returned to normal and my symptoms have never returned.

- In another situation, I injured my back transferring a patient and any movement would send excruciating spasms radiating through my lower back. Again, I was prescribed opiates, Flexeril, hot and cold packs, and was referred to physiotherapy. After months of this not working, I choose to picture the pain as a good thing and attributed it to my kundalini energy rising. It wasn't long before my symptoms subsided. By applying new meaning to my situation, the belief in energy, and the power of my mind, I transformed my condition into something positive. We have the ability to choose with the power of free will, the words and actions we will take in any given situation.

In all of these situations, it was the power of the mind that shifted the energies, allowing for a healing event to occur. In order for lasting change to happen, a new behavior or thought pattern must become a habit to make it stick. That is why those who have had miraculous recoveries and go back to their same way of thinking and doing things, find that their condition returns. Awareness is the key to change. Attention grows things. Therefore, concentrate on what you want, not on what you don't want. The body is very obedient, so it is important that you do not criticize. It is now the time to move away from self-hate, fear, and guilt to self-love, compassion, and approval of yourself.

The energy of a new realization or the 'aha' moment shifts the current expression and resolves the blocks (and therefore, the dis-ease)—a quantum leap. This is due to downward causation, where all that is physical was once a thought or intention. Thoughts are things and thoughts create the chemical processes within your body and in your perceived reality, as well as out to the Universe activating the Law of Attraction. The first law of healing is, "As he thinketh within himself, so is he" (Proverbs 23:7). Quantum physics proves that observation changes the way particles (electrons) act and has been scientifically repeated with the double-slit experiment.

"Live life in the present moment and be aware of the opportunities that present themselves in the wave of possibilities."
(Dr. Robin J. Lambrecht, 2016).

- Namaste -

About the Author

Dr. Robin J. Lambrecht, I-MD

As is often the case, it was my own struggles as well as those of my family (heart disease, cancer, autoimmune disease) that lead me on this path. I successfully recovered from chronic fatigue, colitis, back injury, polyarthritis, and reversed my hypothyroid condition as well as chronic hives, and now I am passionate about helping others obtain optimal health. If you decide that you want to address your emotional toxicity, let me know.

Robin has 30 years of experience working in the healthcare field, both in conventional and natural medicine. She has been awarded World Leader in Health Care by the International Nurses Association for her innovative PTSD treatment involving the subconscious mind. Dr. Robin is the recipient of the ARNET award for outstanding education and practice.

Robin has a Doctorate & PhD in Integrative Medicine (I-MD), a Doctor of Natural Medicine (DNM), a Doctor of Humanitarian Services (DHS), a Master Herbalist and is a Karuna Ki Master Reiki practitioner and teacher. She has a master's degree in nursing.

She has been an instructor for St. John's Ambulance for over 10 years and taught the Nursing Baccalaureate Degree Program in collaboration with the University of Alberta. She is a Certified Distance Education Instructor (CDEI).

She wrote a Practitioner Spotlight blog for Explore Holistic on anger management. She also wrote a holistic article monthly for a local magazine, Just Hers from inception to completion and has been published in Education Resource for a hydration program she co-developed for the Health Region in Alberta.

Dr. Lambrecht has taught on many health topics over the years and has been a keynote speaker on empowerment for the Dental Association. Robin continues to teach through developing courses and writing blogs, articles, PDFs and books.

Stopping the body's signals with medication, cutting out diseased or blocked organs, or radiating tissue to stop growth does not deal with the reason it is happening—the root cause. Until you deal with the reason for your disease, it will continue to present and progress into further body damage. Everything is intertwined—we must treat all five bodies of consciousness to affect a healing response.

Her key role is to support the achievement for self-care through empowerment with real knowledge to apply to health and global policy. It is a new time, a new science, a new paradigm for holistic health and wellness. Start your journey today.

Visit www.QuantumBioHealth.com for more information.

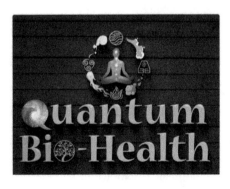

HEALING: WHERE THE FREQUENCY MATTERS

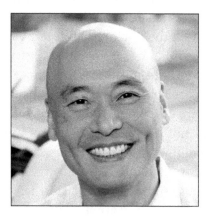

Dr. Jyun Shimizu

On what had seemed so far like an ordinary Monday morning, I was getting ready to see my first patient. As I was leaving my office to walk into the treatment room, I heard my phone vibrate. I quickly glanced at the screen, planning to call back at my first opportunity. I saw my brother's name appear on the call display. He hadn't called me once since I had moved to the US years prior. Although I was initially puzzled, this feeling quickly changed into this inner knowing of "this can't be good news." Sure enough, my brother's first words were, "Mother is in trouble."

I immediately felt a jolt running through me from head to toe, as I had just been hit by lightning. He continued, "She has been sick for the last couple weeks and started to cough up blood. According to the doctors at the hospital, she has an acute infection of some sort. She was admitted to the Emergency Room and is now in the ICU." I could sense a myriad of emotions starting to rise within but tried as good as I could to remain calm.

Within seconds, I felt my role shift from that of a son and brother to that of a doctor and started to evaluate the medical situation.

My brother explained, "The X-ray image displays a shadow that looks like a hole in her esophagus located next to a major artery. If the infection moves from the esophagus to the artery, it will spread through her body very quickly. She could die from the shock of infection. That is the physician's best guess." I hung onto his every word, my brain fixating on one phrase in particular, "What do you mean 'a shadow that looks like a hole?'" I asked.

He replied, "Well, the doctors said it is a vague image. They think it could be a hole, but maybe not. But without a doubt, there is something very unusual in the image." He continued, "The team of physicians gave us two options. If we do surgery to remove her entire esophagus, we may be able to save her life. However, she will not be able to talk or eat anymore. She will need to be tube-fed. If we don't do the surgery and there is a hole, then she could die from an infection."

These were daunting facts. A decision needed to be made, but all these uncertainties were making it impossible. How do you make a decision based off of so many uncertainties? Unfortunately, my mother's story is not a rarity. In such dire situations, many people make fear-based decisions, opting for surgery, hoping to avoid the ultimate pain of losing their beloved. Instead, I took a moment to gain perspective. We knew for sure, from tissue cultures, saliva, and blood samples, that she was indeed fighting multiple bacterial and viral infections. However, the physician's suggestion for surgery was based on an assumption from a vague X-ray image. I asked my brother that the mother be kept on IV medication until I get there and hopped on the next flight to Tokyo.

On my flight from Seattle to Tokyo, difficult though it was, I tried to keep my mind quiet and focused on positive thoughts. When I finally arrived in the ICU, I found my mother hooked to countless hospital gadgets, looking weak and delicate. The last time I had seen my mother, she was vibrant, smiling, and happy. Seeing her so frail made my heart feel tight and heavy. As I approached her bed, she slowly opened her eyes. Her vitality was weak. We spoke briefly, and then I began my work to investigate her condition further. Through communication with my mother's cells using frequency-based testing, I was able to confirm there was no hole in her esophagus. Collective inventories of which modalities, energetic medicine, and applications were needed to restore harmonic frequencies—or in other words, health— within her body.

What a relief! We had just ruled out the worst-case scenario. I updated the team of physicians overseeing my mother's care with my findings, and we all agreed it was best to continue the IV medications and keep monitoring her condition in the meantime. Over the next couple of days, my mother's fever started to calm down, her vitality returned, and soon the physicians took another X-ray image of her esophagus. Our whole family gathered in my mother's room as they delivered the news that, "The artifact in the image was the shadow of a bubble, not a hole."

Allopathic medicine mostly relies on diagnostic tools that provide information on the physical body at a specific point in time. CT scans, ultrasounds, MRI, blood scans, as well as indicators from blood tests, EEG, EKG, NCV tests, and so on, are limited when it comes to viewing smaller than the cellular level. In other words, Western medicine is based on Newtonian physics, the study of mechanics and mass, which used to be our theory to explain the Universe. Newtonian physics is no longer a wholly encompassing explanation for the Universe; the leading theory is quantum physics, which is a new branch of science, is an explanation on how sub-atomic particle (subtle energy) behave. Atoms make the molecule, the molecule makes the cell, and the cells build organs and tissue. Atoms can even be further broken down and observed as sub-atomic particles made of energy.

Nikola Tesla has famously said, "If you want to find the secrets of the universe, think in terms of energy, frequency, and vibration." Frequency carries information that is very specific to each atom, cell, tissue, and organ. It is the mediator between the energy field and physical body. Through Frequency Specific Resonance, it became possible to communicate with the body, the cells, and tap in their innate memory to discover "the story," which leads to the physical and emotional expression as signs and symptoms. At an atomic level, it may be difficult to comprehend this idea in general, but most people are aware of how frequency impacts their body in daily life. For instance, would you put your head next to a microwave? Do you wear a lead vest while getting x-rayed? Would you rather be in the same room with someone happy or upset? When you're angry, does your pet come to you or avoid you?

Energy and frequency may sound like New Age thinking, but it is a well-known fact that all colors, sounds, and words are frequencies. In fact, our survival is closely linked to our ability to interpret the frequencies of all kinds. There are many frequencies that we are impacted by or utilize daily: radio waves, cell phone signals, fiber optic cables, home lighting, and even sunshine. All frequencies influence our cells, whether positively or negatively, and as a result, we can experience great vitality or dis-ease.

Dr. Bruce Lipton explains in his book, The Biology of Belief, epigenetics, that our cells have a memory and that our environment can impact our DNA expression. Independent of the brain, the body will react purely based on memory and environmental stimuli. Environmental stimuli are not limited to what you eat and where you sleep, it can be the thoughts you think, how you are spoken to, and how you perceive your life.

In 2018, IKEA conducted an experiment called "Bully A Plant" to show how destructive negative comments can be. Two identical plants were set up in a school in, and students were instructed to speak positive affirmations to one of the plants, such as "I love you," "You are beautiful," and "You are awesome." The other plant received negative comments such as, "I hate you," or "You are ugly." After four weeks, the plant that received positive feedback was thriving, and only a couple feet away, its counterpart that was spoken to negatively was visibly dying.

Dr. Masaru Emoto, the pioneer of water research worldwide, proved that water molecules were impacted by sound, color, words (intention), and energy and would create unique crystal formations as a result of these influences. Water collected from pure, natural sources, blessed by priests, and given good intention all displayed symmetrical crystalline structure when frozen. Water from disposable plastic bottles, exposed to dissonant music or treated poorly, all revealed distorted structures when frozen.

Dr. Emoto's work proved that water is highly influenceable and can retain memory. This discovery gives new meaning to the fact that our body is made of 62–65% water, and the brain and heart are 73% water.

From the above, you can see how your voice, intention, and words have information. If everything complies with frequency, the language of the Universe, then cells have memory and can communicate what happened to them through resonance. Frequency is what communicates, what happened to the water, what happened to the cell, and at the end, frequency is the mediator between the information field and our bodies. Frequency is information. If a specific frequency is applied to the cell, and it resonates with that frequency, it is a strong confirmation that frequency or information is true. It is with this knowledge and these techniques that I was able to assess and treat my mother.

Imagine the outcome if we had opted to remove her esophagus based on unnerving findings offered by one-dimensional diagnosis and our minds, heart, and judgment being under siege. My mother would no longer be speaking to us, nor would she have the ability to eat. Her quality of life would be drastically affected. About a month later, my mother's health had improved enough for her to be able to leave the hospital. My family called shortly after their arrival home. We were all grateful the worst was now behind us. Thankfully, the ability to communicate with my mother's body saved her life.

My family also reported exciting news regarding my father. During my visit to Japan, I had also used the Frequency Specific Resonance Technique to get to the bottom of a nagging knee pain that had rendered him inactive and consequently led to an overall decline in his health. Once I discovered the "why" behind the pain, I was able to apply the appropriate treatment modalities, which led to stellar results, as opposed to simply treating the symptom like inflammation, decreased mobility, and pain. My brother was excited to report that my father had begun walking miles and miles without any pain! He had also started going to the gym, lifting weights, and swimming for hours daily. My father became so motivated due to his body's transformation that he began to study nutrition, training, and kinesiology.

Fast-forward nine years, my mother is now 76 years old, active, healthy, and happily enjoying her children and grandchildren. My father is now 82 years old, is still going to the gym daily for three hours a day, and very proud to share with others that he has been interviewed on Japanese TV for his accomplishments in the gym. He is a living example of what the human being is capable of.

Among many seemingly miraculous cases, I would like to mention another example to you. A 60-year-old male, Alexander had been battling severe hypertension for the last 25 years. He honestly believed he had spent more than half a million dollars going from one specialist to the other, desperately trying to find a solution to a blood pressure that would regularly go beyond 200/130. Alexander asked that I inquire what the root cause of his hypertension was. To our surprise, we found out that it was related to electromagnetic radiation as a part of significant irritants for this body. I expected Alexander to tell me he had been working in high tech or perhaps in the nuclear industry. No, Alexander shared he was working from a home office but had more electronics in his office than one could imagine possible. As a result, he was literally soaking in toxic EMF all day long. Thinking back, he realized his high blood pressure coincided with the time he had transitioned from being a CEO in the corporate world to having his private consulting business with a home office. To resolve the issue, Alexander needed to make changes in his home office. He invested in proper required devices to shield the EMFs and worked to detox his body of the EMF radiation. His efforts paid off; no more than a week later, his blood pressure had significantly decreased to 130/85 consistently.

Another case involves a 5-year-old boy named Michael, who had behavioral problems. He had a loving and attentive mother, a natural birth, a before-school routine, a healthy diet – everything a child seemingly needs. And yet, Michael had problems with patience, slept unsoundly, and was sensitive to noises, such as the laundry dryer. Testing with the FSR technique indicated that Michael suffered from high levels of EMF toxicity! When I revealed this information to the mother, she was stunned. The

Wi-Fi router for their house was located under Michael's bed and powered on 24/7. I suggested she relocate the Wi-Fi router somewhere else in the house and set up a follow-up appointment four weeks later for Michael. Within a week, we had received a phone call to cancel Michael's appointment; the mother ecstatically reported that he was sleeping soundly throughout the night and was no longer exhibiting behavioral issues at school!

Both of these cases indicate a high sensitivity of the human body to frequencies. Electromagnetic radiation from Wi-Fi routers impacted the bodies of these two very different clients in unique ways. More importantly, both cases demonstrated the willingness of the human body to heal when exposed to the right environment.

We experience that our body is not only the physical body. As a matter of fact, "We are spiritual beings having a physical experience," not the other way around, as quoted by French Philosopher Pierre Teilhard de Chardin. We have an energetic body that supports our physical body. Emotion and energy are intertwined. Our minds give meaning to our feelings. Consciousness is the mediator between our mind and the spiritual body. The increased awareness of quantum physics has brought a scientific awareness of the connection between the spiritual body and the physical body.

Since the discovery of frequencies in the 1900s by many physicists and scientists, including Nikola Tesla, there are many examples of how specific frequencies might cause physical illness. Clear examples of this would be toxic electromagnetic fields from cell signals or nuclear radiation. However, the right frequencies can also restore equilibrium and initiate healing. Remedies, supplements, healer's techniques, and frequency-based medicine and healing will significantly complement the various existing therapeutic and healing methods, including Western medicine. Moreover, when we become co-creators between the healer and patient, we discover new answers to unknown questions. Through the application of resonance frequency, the new paradigm is beginning to unfold for future medicine and healing.

About the Author

Dr. Jyun Shimizu, PhD

Jyun was inspired by his family's value of compassion, a balanced diet, and natural healing in Japan. Following his family background, he pursued Traditional Chinese Medicine in the 1990s. In the 2000s, he expanded his knowledge to homeopathic, natural medicine, and the Bio-energetic field. After 2010, he started to integrate all aspects of medicine and healing into his practice. As of 2020, he has acquired his Doctorate and PhD in Integrative Medicine based on Quantum Principles and is actively applying these principles to clients dealing with chronic illnesses and diseases in his private practice.

He is also the co-founder of ISAMIZU, a global company dedicated to empowering individuals to take control of their health proactively based on the principles of science, consciousness, and technology.

Contact Information:

Websites: www.drjyun.com
www.ISAMIZU.com

THE MIRACLE OF FREQUENCY MEDICINE

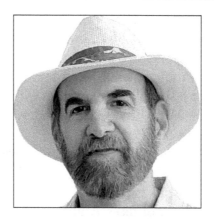

Dr. Steve Small

In the mid 1950s, one of the greatest scientists of the 20th Century, Dr. Albert Einstein stated, "The future of medicine is frequency medicine," and another great scientific genius, Dr. Nikola Tesla remarked in the 1930s, "If you want to find the secrets of the universe, think in terms of energy, frequency and vibration." Why did two of the greatest scientific minds of our century both direct us to focus on the concept of frequency? This is the story of my personal; journey of discovering the greatest Miracle Frequency Healing Device of our time!

I grew up as a kid in the '50s being allergic to everything—cats, dogs, horses, pollen, mold, ragweed, you name it! My mother's cousin was a world-renowned ear, nose, and throat specialist, Dr. Samuel Ganz, an allergist in New York City. As a young child, I would take the subway ride, with my mother, to his office every three months to have my sinuses drained and was ultimately placed on an antihistamine, twice a day, at age seven.

Knowing what I know today, about medication side effects, I am amazed that I was able to actually, stay awake in school. When I graduated the University of Pennsylvania and had the ability to do laboratory testing in my office, I wondered what foods I might be allergic to, as those tests were never performed on me.

As it turned out, the foods at the top of my allergy list were milk and dairy products. I was someone who drank a minimum of a gallon of milk a day. Once I realized that milk was the trigger, I completely eliminated all dairy from my diet. Within a week, I no longer had to go through a box tissues every morning. It was a major life changing experience to understand that to resolve any chronic health condition, one must look at the underlying cause of a disease and not just focus on symptoms with pharmaceutical medication. As obvious as that sounds today, it was a unique approach, back in the late '70s.

As I began my practice in nutritional and preventive medicine in 1978, I decided that every patient, regardless of condition, would undergo a food allergy test. This was my way of focusing on the underlying cause of disease, utilizing a method that was under the control of the patient. We decide what we put into our mouths every day. What I quickly discovered was that by doing food allergy testing, most patient's health issues improved significantly. When you eat a food that you're allergic to, you create an inflammatory response in the body. My primary approach to healing has always been that inflammation is the underlying cause of all disease. Most every chronic disease can be tracked back to inflammation, which can cause autoimmune reactions and lead to degeneration and cancer. The leading contributor of inflammation is stress, so ultimately, one must deal with the stress that causes inflammation in order to reverse it.

In the mid 1980s, I was interviewed for a cover story in Philadelphia Magazine regarding my unique approach. Pat Croce, one of the coaches of the Philadelphia Flyers NHL Hockey team, subsequently asked me if I would be interested in working with the team to help them "get out of last place." The idea was to test the individual players, in my office, so that I could help to optimize their performance on the ice. This was especially important during the third period, when they all ultimately to run out of gas.

Needless to say, after three months of incorporating my recommendations into their daily regimen and eliminating the foods they were allergic to, the Flyers moved into first place! I awoke one morning to see a full-page story in the sports section of the Philadelphia Inquirer newspaper entitled "Murray Craven has the Cow off his Back." He was the Captain of the Flyers. The reporters had been curious to discover how the team was able to rise so quickly from the basement to first place. At a morning practice, the players told them about their treatment with "Doc Steve" and how I had taken them off all the foods they were allergic to. I also recommended some personalized nutritional supplements which together, gave them back the energy they needed to win all of their games. Subsequently, I became a frequent guest on the local Philadelphia CBS News affiliate, KYW-TV, with my weekly nutrition and health segment.

In early 1990, I relocated to Los Angeles after being recruited to be the Director of the University of Santa Monica Center for Health, a multidisciplinary complementary medicine practice. Within a matter of months, A-list celebrities started showing up at my office. I began to work with many of my idols: Steven Spielberg, Sylvester Stallone, Robin Williams, and Britney Spears, to name just a few. In the trade magazines, I began to be referred to as "The Doctor to the Stars," because of my patients in the entertainment, sports, and music industries.

However, unbeknownst to me, my life was about to take a dramatic turn of events. In 1993, after having breakfast with Oscar-nominated actress and close friend, Sally Kirkland, I was involved in a near-fatal car crash when a truck came barreling down Santa Monica Blvd. in West Hollywood and smashed into the driver's side of my sportscar. I remember turning to Sally and saying, "I'm dying," as I felt all the oxygen being sucked out of my body. Fortunately for me, she was able to jump out of her side of the car and have someone call 911.

Fortunately, we weren't far away from Cedars Sinai Medical Center. The next five minutes were a blur, but I distinctly remember hearing what I can only describe as a beautiful chorus of angels and seeing all of the faces of the people in my life flash in front of me, and I wasn't afraid. Simultaneously, I experienced a bright and warm white light encompass me and heard a powerful voice say, "Don't worry, it isn't your time yet. You have lots more to do and many more people to help before it's your turn to leave this plane of existence." The next sound I heard was the ambulance siren and an oxygen mask being placed over my face, just in the nick of time.

At the hospital I was told I had broken all of my ribs, and that my spleen had been ruptured, but I was alive. I spent the next nine days in intensive care and another nine months doing rehabilitation. I had been on a spiritual path since the late '70s, studying under a visionary spiritual teacher named John-Roger with the Movement of Spiritual Inner Awareness. After I was discharged from the hospital, he came to visit me and confirmed that I had indeed had a near death experience. That experience awakened me to the knowledge that we as humans are not bound by the limitations of our five senses. There is more in this world that what we can perceive. We are trained in our society that if we can't see it, feel it, touch it, or hear it, then it doesn't exist. That experience made me aware of the existence of the many realms and dimensions that coexist as one.

A number of years later, I awoke one morning feeling rather bizarre. My entire body was buzzing with what appeared to be an electrical current; it was as if I were plugged into the outlet in the wall. It was completely overwhelming and stayed with me 24/7. I started having very bizarre experiences, seeing auras around people, being able to read people's minds, and other strange phenomena. It felt like I was having, what has been referred to as a psychotic break. I sought the help of my dear friend, Dr. Robert Lawrence, a renowned biochemist and physicist. When I told him what I was experiencing, he briefly left the room and returned with a sheet of paper and said, "Check off all of the experiences you are having right now." I checked off 19 out of the 20 on the list, with which he confirmed, "You are having a Kundalini Awakening Experience." I had no idea at the time to what he was referring. He then added, "Don't worry, it's only a temporary experience. Your body is not able to maintain that amount of energy for an extended period of time and enjoy it while it's happening." He then added, "You're blessed that this has happened to you spontaneously, as it can traditionally take a regular meditator 10 to 20 years to achieve this goal." I had been meditating since the late '70s. I was referred to a researcher at UCLA who had studied Swami Muktananda when he was visiting L.A. He too confirmed, I was having an authentic Kundalini Awakening Experience and that it would eventually leave my system as quickly as it had appeared.

I remember waking up on Day 31 of that experience, standing in the shower and noticing the energy was gone. I wasn't sure whether to be happy or sad. The experiences I had during those 31 days was truly surreal and transformational. There were times strangers would follow me into stores on the streets of L.A. saying things like, "You're a healer and read this verse and this passage from the Bible." I had experiences of time travel. I could make the roses in my garden grow really tall and fast. I could focus on a friend and know exactly where they were and what they were doing at that exact moment. The energy coming out of my hands was always so hot that if I touched a person, it could literally burn them. I've been told that for one person to experience both a near death experience and a Kundalini Awakening is extremely rare, but I came to realize why those two powerful phenomena happened to me. I believe the Universe was revealing to me that there were so many levels of consciousness and awareness beyond our perceived three dimensions. It was this knowledge that became the impetus for my next quantum leap into the miracles of frequency medicine.

On Christmas Eve 1999, while attending an annual seminar lead by my spiritual teacher, I was handed a note saying, "John-Roger wants to see you in his office right away." My first thought was *that's strange timing. I wonder if I've done something wrong.* He had summoned me before he was going onstage and said, "I have some very important information to relay to you. The work you're doing currently in the field of functional medicine is going to completely evolve. You're going to move into a higher realm of healing." It's a realm that he referred to as energy medicine. "You're going to happen upon a very special healing device, that is going to change your life, and how you practice healthcare. You're also going to help a lot of people, using this new technology. Unfortunately, I can't give you the specifics, but you will know when you find it." I was very intrigued and a little confused, but based on past results; he had always guided me to my next steps of my spiritual unfoldment on this level.

Six months later, I was appearing as a guest on a television talk show about anti-aging medicine. After the conclusion of the show, the host pulled me aside and said, "You're a really cutting-edge guy. I want to share an experience I had recently. I visited the office of a Korean doctor in town and he showed me an amazing new quantum biofeedback device. This device is able to do a complete scan of a person's morphogenic field and treat them using resonant frequencies." I immediately asked for his card and made an appointment to see him. He told me it was manufactured in Europe, by a quantum physicist who had worked at NASA on the Apollo Space Program. I immediately sensed that this was the healing device that my spiritual teacher had "seen" and I called the company and asked if their representative would be willing to fly out to Los Angeles so I could test it out on a few of my patients.

Being a research-oriented guy, I wanted to put this new mysterious device to the test before spending $20,000, which was the average price of those types of devices at the time. They now can cost as much as $40,000 in 2020. I told them would be bringing along three patients that had very unique medical conditions. They could run a scan on all three and without asking any questions or gathering any info, they were to present me with a report that detailed their specific health conditions and a treatment protocol. One patient had been born in Ukraine near Chernobyl when he was a child and had been exposed to a lot of nuclear radiation before coming to the U.S. Another person had a congenital heart defect. The third person was dealing with adult attention deficit disorder. To my amazement and fascination, the reports were 100% accurate. I purchased the device on the spot and was told that I was one of the first doctors in the U.S. to have the device. About a week later, it arrived from Europe and I immediately called my spiritual teacher. "Remember that special healing device you told me about six months ago? I just received it." He responded, "Bring it over to my house now." I hooked him up and began the scan, and he confirmed, "This is it. This is what I saw."

This device was one of the very first quantum biofeedback devices that were available at that time, and I was blessed to be one of the first doctors in the U.S. to actually get my hands on one. Currently, it is still the main device that I use in my practice to this day and it's never been wrong. With this device, I am able to determine within minutes the nature of their underlying condition. It also guides me on which specific protocols to use, to help bring their body back into balance on the physical, mental, and emotional levels. It allows me to analyze a patient in a way that cannot be accomplished with traditional laboratory bloodwork.

We live in a world where everything is ultimately composed of energy and frequencies. We are electrical beings. Einstein's Theory of Relativity, E=MC2 applies in every condition and circumstance. Mass equals energy. Our bodies are composed of atoms and molecules and the space in between. We are all connected to the greater information field, where everything inter-relates. It's referred to in physics as quantum entanglement. This leads me, dear reader, to the dream I've had for over the past 10 years. The discovery of what I believe is the next paradigm shift in healthcare and a true miracle of healing.

Ever since I started using my quantum resonant frequency device during the past 20 years, I dreamt of a time when I would have a portable frequency device that I could give to my patients. When they left my office, they would be able to continue using the balancing treatments I had begun. The device had to be affordable to the masses, easy to operate by the layman, and have the capability of scanning and balancing in real time and be specific to the individual. During my career, I have studied and practiced the concepts of intention and manifestation. I have been able to connect to the universal information field, the virtual library of past, present, and future events we all have access to and bring forward my dreams and aspirations. One thing I have learned over the years is that the more specific you are in your request, the more likely you will be to succeed in receiving the outcome you desire.

For example, many patients have spoken to me about wanting to find their ideal relationship. I usually give them a simple homework assignment: Take a pad and write down the 100 qualities you desire in a partner. The most important instruction is to be as specific as you can in your list. This means that it can be the color of the person's eyes, how tall they are, how much money they make, what religion they are, etc. List whatever is important to you, regardless of how mundane it may seem. That person you desire is out there, waiting for you and the Universe now knows exactly who you are looking for. In my manifestation, I was very specific as to the parameters mentioned above. I even added that it would be manufactured in Germany, knowing they make the best frequency devices, and that it wasn't already available in the U.S. I then let it go, with no attachment to the outcome.

Seven days later, that device showed up in my information field! Late one night in November 2019, I was doing some research on the internet, going down the rabbit hole and an interesting site suddenly appeared in German. I thought to myself, "Could this be what I've been dreaming about, all these years? Since I do not speak German, I ran the site through Google Translate. There was no contact info, except for a name and photo. I then searched the name in Google and Facebook. I wrote a text saying, "I'm a doctor in the U.S. that specializes in the field of frequency medicine and I'm interested in distributing your device in the U.S. Within 24 hours, I got a call from a Mr. CJ Peters in Europe, letting me know that he worked with the company and that they were just getting ready to market the device in the U.S. He was especially interested in working with someone who had extensive experience in frequency medicine and in a few days, I received this device, called the Healy in the mail. Now it was time for the ultimate test, just like I done 20 years ago. Could it do what he said it could do?

Here's where we connect the dots to my amazing adventure. Remember the near fatal car accident I had in 1993 at the beginning of my story? What I didn't mention, was that this accident left me with a severe chronic condition, peripheral neuropathy in my right foot. I've lived with this condition for almost 30 years now. Regardless of what treatment I've tried,

I haven't been able to resolve it satisfactorily. If you have or know someone that suffers from this inflammatory condition, it is extremely painful is present 24/7, and makes it extremely difficult to stand on hard surfaces or take long walks. In addition to this, for the last year and a half, I have been unable to drive my car due to loss of proprioception in my right foot. I was unable to quickly move my foot from the gas pedal to the brake and it sometimes got "lost in the air." Besides the extreme anxiety it created while driving, I narrowly missed getting into four separate car accidents! Once, almost careening off of a third story parking garage because I almost couldn't sense the brake pedal in time. At that point, I knew it was not worth getting myself killed in another car accident. So, I relied on friends, Ubers, and Lyfts to get around town. I also lost a sense of independence.

Now was the time for the ultimate test. Could it deliver as promised? So that evening, I hooked myself up to the Healy portable frequency microcurrent device I had just received from Germany. After using it to run two nerve-related frequency microcurrent programs lasting approximately 1.5 hours for three nights in a row, I awoke on the fourth day without any pain in my right foot. Not only that, I was able to take a shower standing on my tiled shower floor for more than five minutes. It usually felt like I was standing on hot coals. Only three days in a row of treatment with the Healy, and my almost 30 years of severe peripheral neuropathy had resolved! On the fourth day, I called up a friend and asked if he would accompany me in the passenger car for a drive. Lo and behold, I was able to drive 20 minutes to brunch and home without any difficulty at all. Today, it's been six months since that fateful day I received my Healy. I no longer am experiencing neuropathy and I am driving normally by myself. I consider this technology to be a game changer in the field of self-care. It's going to allow people to take back responsibility for their own health.

The Healy is an amazing healing tool, not only because it gives us the ability to scan our morphogenetic field, but also balances us through access to 144,000 unique frequencies that are selected using artificial intelligence. Other frequency devices take a more cookbook approach. They use the same fixed frequencies every session to balance a health condition and every person uses those same frequencies The Healy uses a dynamic frequency approach in a secure, encrypted medical cloud in Germany. Every treatment is unique for that person, at that moment in time. The microcurrent allows us to raise the cell membrane potential to -70mv, the level of a young, healthy cell. As the cell voltage drops, cells become inflamed, create tumors, and ultimately die.

Another exciting aspect of the Healy is its ability to deliver electroceuticals directly into our cells. Over the past six months, electroceuticals have been referred to as the future of medicine in publications like Scientific American and Time magazine. It's a brand new medical technology that allows us the ability to deliver substances like medications and chemotherapy, directly into the cells of the body, bypassing the gastrointestinal tract and thereby eliminating side effects. Healy has an electroceutical program that can deliver the frequencies of vitamins, minerals, amino acids, and hormones directly into our body, achieving 100% absorption in the cell, as opposed to only 10% through oral ingestion. The frequencies direct the microcurrent, like the driver of a car, to their appropriate destinations inside the body.

I believe that everything in life happens for a reason and that everything we experience is an extension of the information field, the virtual library of past, present, and future events we all have access to. When I think back over all the experiences I have been through over the past 40 years, it is easy to see how each event led me to my next level of unfoldment. The car accident, the near-death experience, the neuropathy, and the Kundalini Awakening were all connected events in the information field. Those experiences have led me to where I am today. Being given the opportunity to connect into other dimensions of reality opened the doorway to knowing that we are not bound by our five senses alone. There are many additional dimensions in our Universe we can explore. Using a frequency microcurrent device such as the Healy on a daily basis, you can connect directly to the information filed and allow your body to heal itself. By providing us with the correct frequencies our body needs, it becomes the ultimate Miracle of Healing.

About the Author

Dr. Steve Small

Dr. Steve Small received his B.S. in Biology and B.A. in Psychology from the State University of New York, Stony Brook. He earned his DMD from the University of Pennsylvania and received his postgraduate N.M.D. (Nutritional Medicine) and O.M.D. (Orthomolecular Medicine) degrees. In 1981, Dr. Small opened the Center for Well Being, the first holistic health center on the East Coast.

In 1990, Dr. Steve relocated to Los Angeles to become Director of the University of Santa Monica Center for Health, a complementary medical practice. He is frequently referred to as the "Doctor to the Stars" in the media because of his high-profile practice where he treats many members of the film, television, music industry, and professional sports community.

Dr. Steve is a frequent guest on radio and TV and has had own weekly health talk show on Sirius Satellite Radio. He lectures to doctors and health practitioners around the world and has been the keynote speaker at the International Bioenergetic Medicine Conference in 2005 in Budapest, Hungary, 2006 Rosarita Beach, Mexico, 2007 Cancun, Mexico, 2008 Amsterdam, Netherlands, 2009 Budapest, Hungary, 2016 Athens, Greece and Budapest, Hungary 2017, as well as in San Diego for the Institute of Stress Sciences. In 2013, Dr. Small received the Nelson Medicine Award in recognition of his Excellence in Energetic Medicine. Dr. Steve is currently the Director of Quantum Health in Los Angeles, where he practices quantum energetic and frequency medicine. He is also the Dean of the International Medical University of Natural Education, N.A. and serves as a Member of the HealyWorld Product Board and Healy USA Mastermind Group.

Contact Information:

Email: healydocsteve@gmail.com
Phone: 888-HEALYUS
www.healyworld.net/en/partner/DocSteve

TAKING CHARGE: THE MIRACLE OF GROUNDING

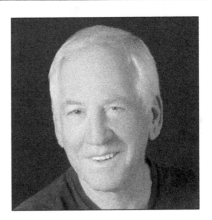

Clint Ober

The miracle is of myself having spent 30 years in the communications industry, having no knowledge or real background in biology and health, although I did grow up on a ranch and spent a lot of time around animals and caring for their health. I grew up in an agricultural/animal husbandry type background, and I was considered a cowboy by my grandfather. What we looked for is any animal in the herd that didn't look like the rest.

In my youth I took a big interest in television spent 30 years in the communications industry as one of the people who helped pioneer many aspects of it. As we developed the cable system, we learned that you had to ground everything because there were miles of metal cable up in the air. You had to ground it to the earth because of the wind will blow, creating static electricity, or because of lightning. As long as we did everything perfectly, they would get a nice, clear sound, nice, pretty picture.

Most people do not understand what ground is, other than it is the earth that we're standing on. The ground is an electrical phenomena, meaning that one surface of the earth, it has a negative surface charge. This means there's an abundance of electrons that immediately move and reduce positive charge. If you walk across a carpet with rubber shoes, you build up a static charge. If you touch something metal, sometimes you'll feel the shock but there's always a discharge there.

I became very sick when I was 50 and was just going downhill more and more every few days. I went to the doctor and learned that I had a major abscess in my liver. They drained it right there on the spot and the next morning the infectious disease doctor said, "Well, we have some good news and some not so good news." The good news was that they had figured out what was wrong with me. The bad news was that I needed surgery immediately. They performed an experimental surgery to cut out as much of the liver as they possibly could (where the abscess was) and see what effect it had. Of the six pockets the liver has, they cut out five of them. I didn't know what to expect, nor did I have any choice. The night before the surgery, I was in immense pain. The next thing I knew a couple of days later, I woke up in the ICU. After that, I went home after a week or so and slowly recovered. About six months later, my liver had grown back 100%.

Ultimately, I survived but as I started to accept all of this, I hadn't gone back to work. I owned a company that had hundreds of employees and lived on a mountaintop in a 5,000 square foot A-frame. But I kept looking around and I realized that I almost died, and what would have happened to all these things? It was quite disturbing to me that I had spent my whole life collecting all of these things and I had made my life about this. I had this thing go through me that I didn't want to own anything. Then, I bought a small RV and took two and a half suitcases of clothing and personal things and hit the road. I spent four years driving around the United States and visiting my children. I didn't want to make my life about money any longer and I didn't want to be responsible for anyone else. I gave the company to the employees and spent a lot of time in RV parks and being close to nature because that's where I felt the best.

I stood outside of my RV one night and witnessed a beautiful sunset. This vibrancy came to life and I remember that feeling that came over me, like the earth was talking to me. That would be natural, because where I grew up, Native Americans said that everything is connected. A blade of grass is your cousin; everything is one, and you're a part of it – not apart from it. I had this feeling and felt that I had to do something. I went in the RV that night and I wrote on a piece of paper:

"Become an opposite charge."

To me, that meant going out and stirring people up, poking them, charging them up – probably from my cowboy days. Then I wrote a second line:

"Status quo is the enemy."

I had no idea what it meant.

The next morning, I decided to go back West. I ended up in San Diego and didn't feel right, so I turned around and went back to Tucson. I didn't feel right still, so the next morning I decided to drive to Flagstaff, because that is similar to where I'm from in elevation and nature. It was getting very late and I saw a sign before going up the hill to Flagstaff that pointed to an RV park in Sedona. No one was there, so I just pulled in and plugged in. I woke up the next morning, looked outside, and said, "I'm not leaving here." It felt like the right place, and I ended up staying two years.

One day when I was in Sedona, I wanted to use my computer, but it kept crashing. I realized there was static electricity on my body that caused it to happen. I laid a piece of metal tape across the desk in front of the computer, connected it to a wire, and then connected it to an electrical ground. Before I touched the computer, I would touch the tape first, solving the problem of the static charges.

About a half hour later, a tour bus with a bunch of Japanese tourists pulled up. The only thing I noticed was their white tennis shoes. I intuitively asked myself, "I wonder if there is a problem with humans no longer being grounded because now, we wear these rubber-soled shoes?" That night, I took out an alternator and connected it to a ground rod in the yard. Then, I started walking around the house with the wire and measuring the charges on my body as I wasn't grounded versus when I took my shoes off and stood barefoot outside. The largest amount of environmental noise from static and EMF was in my bedroom. Have you seen sparks in your bedding sometimes? I suspected this could be a problem. I went to the hardware store and bought a roll of metalized duct tape, what you would normally put around heating vents. I laid it across the bed, connected it to a wire with an alligator clip, and ran the wire out to connect it to a ground rod.

I lay down on the tape and then I would touch the alternator, so I could see that I was grounded, meaning I had no charge—I was at earth potential. When you touch the earth, your body is negatively charged, meaning you can't have any charge in your body. I dealt with widespread body pain and would go outdoors and ask, "God, why did you make my body with so much pain in it?" That particular night, I had the meter on my chest and watched TV at the foot of the bed. The next morning I woke up and the TV was still on, with the meter lying by my side. I had fallen asleep—and slept all night.

This was remarkable because I hardly ever slept throughout the night, often needing medication to sleep. I tried this on a couple of friends. The next day, one of them said it felt good and thought it helped with sleep. A couple of days later, the other guy came along and asked, "Is there any chance this could have anything to do with arthritis? Because my pain is way down." I realized my pain was also significantly reduced, so there had to be something to this. Later, I researched what I could about grounding and pain, but couldn't find anything. So, I ended up going down to the University of Arizona in Tucson, asking a couple of people down there about the cause of pain, because what I had discovered makes the pain go away.

Back then, if you asked about the cause of conditions like lupus and arthritis, the cause was unknown. Even today, if you look at the cause of MS, the medical cause is unknown. I spoke with some people in the sleep lab and relayed what I had experienced. Well, they thought I was nuts. They did not understand anything about electricity, and I certainly did not understand anything biometrically, so there was a barrier.

But I was insistent because a lot of people are in pain and they can't sleep. Because nobody else wanted to touch the topic, I ended up having to do the first study by myself with the help of a couple of university students and a nurse. I was getting my haircut one day and I heard a couple of the ladies talking about pain and sleep. Bingo! I spoke with the owner and told her about the study. We found 60 people in no time! Half were to be grounded, and the rest were placebo grounded. We made a pad that was one foot wide by two feet long out of conductive material and we would connect it to a ground wire with an alligator clip and connect it to a ground rod outside the bedroom window.

One day, I had these two people. One of them was an elderly gentleman probably in his 80s. He had all kinds of health disorders. I went in and I had him sit on his bed and I measured the static charge on his body and the electromagnetic fields that were on his body. I had assumed at the time that it was because of electrical noise. He lived in an adobe home with an earthen floor. He had a metal bed and no lamps or anything electrical near his bed. He only had one light in the room. I thought it was really unfortunate that he got a live pad, because he had a clean bedroom environment.

That afternoon, I went over to see a woman in her 80s who had fluttering arthritis in both wrists and couldn't hold things in her hands. She sat on the bed and I measured the electric fields in her home, and she had the highest electric fields in her home because of heating pads, lamps, and the sort. The electric fields in case were so high, the ground pad wasn't sufficient to eliminate the charge. I didn't know what kind of results we were going to get with this woman.

It always seemed like the right information showed up at the right time, like there's a hidden hand. While looking at the data about a month later, I knew there was something really wrong. This gentleman had no results. He had no environmental electrical stress and he had no static electricity, yet he had great results. The lady who had so much electrical noise in her home that I couldn't ground it out, her results were phenomenal. They slept better, they felt better, and had less pain. I learned that it's the earth itself. I thought it was grounding out the electrical environment and all the static. But it was the negative surface charge of the earth; as soon as you ground, your body becomes negative. I had this ah-ha moment that the reason we ground everything electric in your home is to maintain electrical stability and prevent fire.

The human body is the most electrical thing in our environment. Every cell in the body is electrical. All of the communications in the body are electrical. By grounding the body, what we're doing is preventing charge within the body and quieting the environmental noise. I knew then that it was the earth itself that produced the results, not all the things I had originally started off with.

About a month or two later, I went down to San Diego and met with a doctor who wanted to learn more about what I was doing, and we designed a new study. We grounded a group of people, so they were their own controls. This time, we measured cortisol for 24 hours and sent it to a lab, and then we grounded them for six to eight weeks. At the end of the study, we measured their cortisol again for 24 hours and sent it to the lab. When I put the participant profiles together in a uniform graph, we saw that all the circadian cortisol profiles synchronized, meaning at midnight they were the lowest and increased by 4:00 a.m., peaking at 6:00 a.m. Afterward, they would slowly drift down for the rest of the day. Cortisol is a master hormone in charge of fight-or-flight, and we recognized that we were normalizing circadian cortisol secretions. In the control, everybody's cortisol looked like spaghetti but after they were grounded, they all synchronized about the same. The ones who had high cortisol came down and the ones who had lower cortisol rose.

There was no environmental cue or clock to tell the body that it was time for cortisol levels to increase. Three of the participants didn't end up finishing because they were stewardesses. Their cortisol was off three hours because their bodies were on New York time. When you're connected to the earth and its electrical field (electrical pulses) the earth absorbs and recognizes the amplitude of the electrical field. It's a cueing mechanism and is what causes cortisol to start increasing at 4:00 a.m. Jet lag happens because your cortisol is off. But if you just go stand barefoot on the earth for 15 minutes, then your body will biologically reset to the earth's circadian rhythm.

Dr. Steven Sinatra, a cardiologist, is someone else we visited. We grounded him and a bunch of other doctors, and they were fascinated. Dr. Sinatra looked at me and he said, "Clint, if you're affecting pain, you need to be researching inflammation, because pain is a byproduct of inflammation. You can't have pain unless you have inflammation first." At this point in 2002, nobody really knew about inflammation. It wasn't in much of the medical literature, either. In 2004, Time magazine featured "Body on Fire." The authors stated that we don't have cancer, this or that; what we have is chronic inflammation, which will manifest differently in people. For some, it will manifest as lupus, MS, arthritis, or cardiovascular disease. In others, it will be cancer.

When you have an injury or pathogen in the body, neutrophils will be sent by the immune system to encapsulate the pathogen or damaged cell, and it will release what's called reactive oxygen species. These are electrically charged molecules that are considered "hot." What they will do is rip the electrons from the pathogen or the damaged cell and destroy it. That's how the immune system works. This is the innate immune system.

In 1960, we invented plastics. The first thing we did is we put them on the soles of shoes. Ninety percent of the visits to the doctor back in 1960 were for infectious disease, childbirth, and acute injury. Ninety-five percent of all visits to a doctor today are for stress-related health disorders and autoimmune disease, meaning the immune system is oxidizing tissue. It doesn't have enough redox potential in the body, meaning there's not enough molecules that can reduce the reactive oxygen species, a free electron. If there's not enough redox, then if there are any of these molecules left over after they have reduced the pathogen, then they will attack an adjacent cell in nanoseconds and steal an electron from it, damaging the cell. The collateral damage from the immune response. That cell screams out to the immune system that something is damaging it and another neutrophil comes and cleans that up. That is how the body catches fire, otherwise known as chronic inflammation.

The immune system now spends most of the time fighting the fire that it itself is creating. But as soon as you ground the body for five or 10 minutes, the pain will stop. You cannot have inflammation in the body when it is grounded. When you go back to 1960, we were either barefoot or wore leather soled shoes. Consider the animal world. The animals that live in the wild do not have cancer, chronic pain, or inflammation-related conditions. But on the other hand, animals that live indoors manifest the same health disorders as their human owners.

Generally speaking, even a half hour of grounding is lifechanging for some people. For others, they have so much damage that it takes a few days or weeks for the body to totally recover. But the thing that we learned is that when you get back to basics by grounding, walking barefoot, and eating live food, the body will return to normal because it doesn't know anything else. That's a big thing to grasp. It doesn't need all of these things that we do, because most of them create more problems than they solve. Our bodies evolved in a grounded environment, and we lost that 60 years ago when we started wearing shoes. Inflammation disorders skyrocketed once we started doing that.

There is another important component to all of this. One day when I was grounding a woman who had severe MS and I asked her how she developed it. She had never thought about it, but about six months prior to developing MS, her mother had died, she went through a divorce, and I lost something dear to her. I got into the habit afterward of asking people with chronic health disorders about their personal history. Every person described a story of loss.

Back when I watched cows, there would be an explosion of jackrabbits some years and coyotes to hunt them. When a rabbit sees the coyote, his ears will spring up and he will jump 10 feet in the air, zigzagging back and forth. The coyote will follow him and almost all of the time will run out of energy. He will lie on the ground panting. The rabbit will run just a little bit further so he can still keep an eye on the coyote, and then will sit there, quivering. All of the sudden, the rabbit will have a big shake and then go back to eating grass like nothing ever happened.

The rabbit is naturally grounded. What happened was as soon as the coyote attacked, the rabbit's cortisol spiked, giving him the energy to run for his life. When it was over, his body was full of inflammation and charged with cortisol. As soon as he was grounded after a moment, he drained it away and when it was gone, shook it off and went back to normal life, eating grass and waiting for the next coyote attack.

With loss, like the rabbit, people (especially the women I treat) go into a fight-or-flight stage because of panic, especially with grief. Some never come out of it, and that's what causes oxidation in the body. When these women were grounded, all of a sudden, they started coming back to life and improving, just like the rabbit. There are countless 'coyotes' all day long that cause cortisol spikes, so they're living at a chronically sympathetic state, but we don't take time to ground it out. If you do nothing more than go outdoors, take a chair, take your shoes off, put your feet in the grass, and just sit there for 30 minutes and let the earth neutralize and discharge all of this inflammation, pain, and stress in your body, then you can go to sleep. Then you can heal and recover and do it all again tomorrow.

Conclusion

We have stepped out of nature. We are a part of the earth and as long as being outside connects us to it, eating its food, we're alive. But as soon as that electricity is gone, we're dead. The miracle is that I was 54 at the time I made these observations. However, I wasn't the first; many generations prior had known about it but forgot the benefits of grounding. I assumed academia and the experts knew everything about any given topic. I've always had the common sense that I call "cowboy logic." I've always been attuned to nature and there's always been this intuitive awareness that speaks to me. I listen and observe but when I don't know when I'm doing, I try to find the expert in the field to fill me in.

There are close to eight billion people on the planet and I get to be the one to ask the question and make my life about something bigger than making money and running a business.

When you come close to death, you look back at your whole life real quick. I was given a second chance and I look at everything differently today. I want to be of service and help as much as I can, but most of all, I want to go to my grave next time knowing personally I'm happy with myself because I made my life about something worthwhile.

About the Author

Clinton Ober

Clinton Ober is CEO of Earth FX Inc., a research and development company located in Palm Springs, California. He first learned of grounding when installing cable TV systems in Billings, Montana in the early 1960s. A decade later, he formed Telecrafter Corporation and built it into the largest provider of cable installation services in the United States. This company specialized in proper grounding of cable installations for safety and TV signal stability. In the 1980s, he turned his attention to the developing computer industry and partnered with McGraw-Hill to distribute live digital news services via cable to PCs. This led to the development of the first cable modem and an increased awareness of need for proper system grounding.

Following a health challenge in 1995, he retired and embarked on a personal journey looking for a higher purpose in life. During his travels, he noticed people wearing plastic and rubber-soled shoes that insulate the body from Earth. He wondered if no longer being naturally grounded could affect us. The question led to an experiment that suggested grounding alone reduced chronic pain and improved sleep. Thereafter, he developed a working hypothesis: Earth grounding the human body normalizes functioning of all body systems. (Corollary: The body utilizes the Earth's electrical potential and free electrons to maintain its internal electrical stability for the normal functioning of all self-regulating and self-healing systems.

Over the past 20 years, he has supported a host of research studies (Earthing Institute) that collectively demonstrate that grounding alone reduces inflammation and promotes normal functioning of all body systems.

Contact Information:
Email: Clint.ober@earthfx.net

MY BEAUTIFUL VISITORS

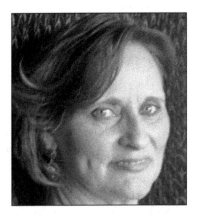

Darla Boone

Let me start by saying that I have had the good fortune in experiencing several amazing spiritual healings and profound out of this world insights throughout my life, miracles you could say. I am usually the one who lands on her feet in life, the one in my family of origin the others, could depend on for advice and help. I love to help people when I can. I am a worldly person, seeker of truth, a visionary, free spirit gypsy soul, independent woman, leader, thinker, researcher, science-minded, and spirit-filled being on a mission. I am also a mother and grandmother. Why am I telling you these things? It's because I want you to have some idea of the kind of person I am so when you read my story about grieving the loss of my sister, Donna, you will better understand what my journey of loss, grieving, healing, and finding a new self might have been like for me.

Maybe you can relate to the feeling of being lost and the joy of being found in the tragedy that happens in life. I think sharing our grief is an integral part of this life journey, and my story may give hope to others. Pain is not something we like to talk about, but it is something we all go through; I am so grateful that God knocked me to my knees. I had nowhere to go except through the pain; I had to let go and let God. And he showed up mightily!

Eighteen months ago, my big Sister Donna passed away unexpectedly and tragically. Six months later, I moved from Palm Springs, California back home to Seattle, Washington. I had lived in California for 25 years, so moving back home was a big decision for me. The Holy Spirit kept encouraging me to go home, whispering in my ear, "You need to be near the water and trees to get grounded, and find your center again," little did I know how important that message was for me, as it may have saved my life. The year of Donna's passing became one of the most challenging years of the experience of my life. Her passing left me feeling extremely traumatized, and because I am a fighter and always on the move, it took time for me to understand just how traumatized I had become.

I now had an enormous hole in my life, energetic field, heart, and faith to heal and fill with something, but I didn't know what. I have been awake spiritually for years and have studied holistic health for years too, and everything in between, but it didn't matter. The impact of my sister's passing surpassed everything I knew; it had changed me at a core level.

I had to grow in ways that I hadn't planned on, and with my busy schedule I had no place to delve into the most profound aspects of self. I needed to accept the unacceptable, to heal, I had to learn a raw new level of understanding about the life, death, forgiveness, love, and the thin veil that separates the living and from those who have passed over. I had to renew myself, and I couldn't fight it. The grief was so deep, there was no escaping the profound physical and emotional impact. I had to enter another spiritual transformation and take a journey without my sister's love and guidance. After all, we were much more than sisters, we were spiritual friends.

Ultimately only myself, my sister, and God/Christ know the real journey I went on, I indeed had to "Let go and let God" and allow myself breakdown so I could breakthrough and step more fully into the person I am to be here on this earth. This became the year of Miracles for me.

I have lost many people throughout my life—as we all have—but losing Donna was a loss that I was entirely not prepared for. Not only were we especially close as sisters and deeply bonded, but also we were friends and spiritual partners, and as the years passed by, we became closer and closer. She was always a presence in my life as I was in hers; we depended on each other, and as all siblings do, we would sometimes disagree. We were both equally opinionated, and even the disagreements were lighthearted.

She struggled with several health issues, both physically and mentally, as well as learning problems that plagued her throughout her life. I, on the other hand, was always healthy, athletic, vibrant, endless energy. Still, Donna's health issues became a highly motivating factor for me to learn how to be of help her, and as a result, I have years of study in the field of Holistic Health and Wellness.

I endlessly tried to find ways to help her deal with health issues from a more holistic and natural approach. Her problems were highly complex because of her mental health issues, and she suffered from multiple personality disorder. It was heartbreaking for me to watch and helplessly try to intervene when we know the prescribed approach for mental illness is heavy medication. But I never gave up, and neither did Donna, in time through her faith and determination and my support, she was able to come off of all medicines except for a small dose of Lithium. She was the strongest person I have ever known; she had tenacity and was a fighter and a winner. Even combating constant health issues and the emotional roller coaster of mental illness she lived with yet was still a profound person; she had a deep sense of her spiritual identity and the courage to face anything. She was my Hero.

Donna passed from a simple fall that happened in her home, a small fracture that landed her in the hospital, and then a skilled nursing facility. They mismanaged of her care, which resulted in her wrongful death, a massive blow for me to overcome. I had spent my life looking out for her, and something so small resulting in her death, even now it is still surreal.

I was extremely traumatized over my sister's passing, and I was there when she passed in the hospital as they tried to save her life. Her passing activated years of suppressed feelings of hurt and loss, of anger and disappointment. This was a pattern that began in my childhood, and those wounds in time became a collective fractal field of trauma that I have lived with and hadn't yet genuinely processed and healed. Neither had my sister; the wounds were a part of our bond.

Her passing caused me to experience a sense of deep separation from everything, even my lofty, even my goals. Donna's passing awakened all of that in me. She was so precious to me, and no other will ever take her place. With all of my power and knowledge, I couldn't save her life. I felt she slipped right through my fingers and that put me on my knees but learning how to grieve her loss changed my life forever and for the better.

After months of the process, a point came where I began to understand what a great and powerful blessing it was for me to go through such personal devastation, which created a tremendous catharsis for me to be set free. I found that no one can tell you how to grieve or for how long. It is our journey, and for me, the whole experience was a Miracle.

Donna was an influential, spirit-filled person in her own right. She had a real connection to God and a personal walk with Lord Jesus. She never ceased to amaze me with profound insight, and she loved her family members and friends deeply. Since her passing she has come to visit me from the other side on several occasions in my dreams and into my room to let me know that she is with me. She has spoken to me through the spiritual realm, but the real Miracle began with an exceptional experience that I had with my sister that shifted my reality about the power of prayer and healing and the other side of the veil.

Some months back I was having a particularly challenging and painful day about the passing of my sister. I was listening to Neil Young's "Harvest Moon," and that song helped me get through the pain of losing Donna. Thank you, God, for music. On this day, I was weeping for her and I was crying out to her, asking her to me let me know she was still here with me in the spirit. I was a mess that day, and I could not be consoled.

My prayers were heard and answered; this was the day that she came to me with Lord Jesus; this was the day that I had powerful spiritual healing and began to heal my deep childhood wounds.

It was an early evening before dark, and it was a beautiful winter sunset in Washington. As an amateur photographer, I decided to take some photos of the sunset. It was cold outside, and I so I went back inside the house and took more pictures through the window. As I began to take more photos, suddenly my phone shut off all by itself and then came back on. I thought that was very strange.

As I looked into the camera lens, to my astonishment this huge orb was dancing around the front yard. I heard my sister say to me, "I am here." I was in overwhelmed and exhilarated all at the same time. I took several pictures of the orb and videotaped for nearly 15 minutes, crying the whole time. And then while standing at the window, I felt my sister standing at my right side and Christ standing behind me.

I heard Donna say, "Darla, you have taken care of everyone your whole life, especially me. You have never let me down. You now have time to heal your inner wounds."

Then I felt the touch of Christ come into mind, and I felt the right and left hemispheres of my brain to begin to tingle. Instantly, I felt my brain go into harmonic aliment and I then felt healing from past childhood memories the internal struggle lift off. At that moment, I knew I had just received powerful spiritual healing from Christ, and I felt a shift and a lightness. It was a beautiful experience and then they were gone.

As the days passed, I notice afterward that I began to pay attention to being more loving to myself, and my higher self has continued to emerge. Magically, my business has continued to grow and expand internationally during this time of great healing. God had given me a vision and a mission for my life many years ago, and the Master Healer released the wrestling match I had been in with my stubborn subconscious in an instant. There has been a lot of letting go of things that no longer serve me or my mission since this healing experience with Christ and my sister. My relationship with my sister has changed, too. I am whole within myself, as she has grown into a vast and powerful angel. I can feel her as I write this to all who read it.

I have many years of scientific research and studying healing and wellness and experiencing profound spiritual insights, so, I thought I understood the elements of trauma. It turns out I didn't. The experience of such a tremendous loss was much different than an intellectual understanding, and my sister became my teacher and healer. That is a Miracle.

I now know something about the word trauma, and it's no match for the power of God's healings for us; you see my mission is to spread this message: *Healing comes from within.* I can never return to the Darla I was before, and that's okay. I am grateful to have the opportunity to still be here in the physical world and to carry my mission forward and share it with the world with my big sister again by my side. I know she is always with me, and I am so grateful for her present.

We live each day as if we will be here forever, because we genuinely are eternal spiritual beings. To me, this is one of God's crazy little mysteries.

About the Author

Darla Boone

Darla is Founder, Executive Producer, and Director of Boone Media International. For the last 12 years, she has been producing PBS Television shows on alternative medicine. These shows include many aspects of healing, wellness, and society, the new paradigm, health science, transformative technology, ancient wisdom, education, green, women, and many other topics.

Boone has entered the path of media in all of its forms along with distribution, marketing, promotion, and sales. She is committed to explore and present through television deeper levels of knowledge and findings in science and in storytelling for the benefit of humanity.

Boone's newest project, "The Potentialist," is a 13-part television episodic series. There is a 30-minute showcase pilot now in preproduction and will launch January 2021 and will air on PBS Television National Broadcast produced under the title Media International in partnership Los Angeles and India Studios.

Contact Information:

Boone Media International
Website: www.boonemediatv.com
Email: darlakboone@hotmail.com
Telephone: 760-699-1705

MIRACLES

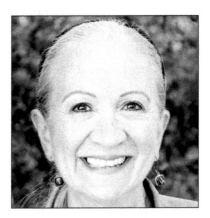

Heather Gunn

Modern medicine's paradigm of disease is based largely upon the eradication of symptoms that simply attempt to tell us that something is wrong, and we continue to shoot the messenger through the use of medications and other interventions, so the underlying message remains unheard. Modern medicine is clearly effective for infectious disease and emergencies; however, it often misses the mark in the treatment of chronic health challenges. After a 40-year nursing career, I firmly believe that we mask the symptoms that carry deeper messages and I have witnessed clear proof that our thoughts, feelings, emotions, and beliefs profoundly affect our health.

The body follows direction from the brain as it releases hormones—chemical messengers produced by the endocrine glands. Hormones are transported by the brain through the circulatory system to regulate physiology and behavior. The major endocrine glands are the pituitary, pineal, thymus, thyroid, adrenal glands, pancreas, testes and ovaries, with each gland corresponding with one of the seven major chakras in the body.

Wake Up: Miracles

Hormones are powerful so too much or too little of a certain hormone can lead to disease.

Sadly, we lose sight of the importance of the patient's belief system in determining recovery from illness. The patient is often conditioned to place a victim-oriented emphasis on the disease rather than on the healing process. Anita Moorjani, best-selling author of *Dying to Be Me and What If This is Heaven*, calls this perspective 'illness scare' rather than 'health care.' Science has shown us that our mirror neurons repeat our experience of an event, so we want that event to be constructive, not destructive. We often fail to connect with our client/patient by failing to open our minds to the potential of the body to heal itself. During my years working in oncology, hospice, rheumatology, ER and OR, I saw firsthand how the connection between mind, body, and Spirit is undeniably key to healing. We must go straight to the deepest seed of the client's emotional, mental, or physical health challenges, which can go as far back as conception or even earlier.

Healing is about moving past confusing messages in the mind by listening to the messages sent through the sensorial intelligence of the body. The body knows how to heal itself; science tells us so. We just need to step aside with patience and unconditional support to give it the opportunity to do so on its own terms. We also need to understand that sometimes healing is not about saving a life. Sometimes it means discovering a deeply personal way to embrace the end of one's life with dignity and grace.

Maria

Maria, a tiny, frail lady in her early '40s, had been undergoing a steady loss of weight and stamina over the past few months. She was diagnosed with Stage 4 inflammatory breast cancer at the clinic where I was working. The red rash surrounding her entire left chest, misdiagnosed as a skin infection, had been treated by her primary physician with antibiotics for several months. Recent testing indicated the cancer was present in most of her lymph nodes and her spine, and her tumor markers were sky-high. She now found herself facing her own mortality.

I was present when the oncologist gave her the dreaded news: her test results indicated a very aggressive cancer. He told Maria

163

that she had maybe three to four months before it would likely claim her life. He explained that aggressive treatment for the cancer would be too much for her frail body to handle. The doctor then stepped out of the room, leaving me to continue the conversation with Maria in terms of her treatment options to assist her to remain comfortable as her cancer progressed.

She was in shock. I sat with her, holding her hands for a few moments. I then asked, "Maria, how do you feel about what the doctor just told you?"

"Feel? How do I feel? I have three children at home..." She was devoid of emotion...utterly still. Fully aware that I was stepping far beyond the usual platitudes spoken at this juncture, I chose to follow my instincts and said to her, "Let me ask you a question...do you want to die, or do you want to live?"

"You mean I have a choice?" Staring at the floor, deeply entrenched in the gravity of her situation, she replied, "Well, I want to live." We then discussed her options. I stressed the importance of connecting with her own Spirit through her heart and allowing it to fill her with hope. I encouraged her to move beyond the situation and ask her own innate wisdom what she needed to do in order to connect her body, her mind and her Spirit.

Three years later, on an unusually warm and sunny early spring day, she located me at the college where I was teaching nursing. With roses and chocolates in hand, she explained that she had decided not to undergo any treatment of any sort, instead opting to place her faith in her deeply religious Christian upbringing. She now had no signs of breast cancer and she appeared healthy and robust. She told me that, through prayer, she became aware that her faith in God was strong, but that her faith in herself was not. "I had always believed that the power to heal lay outside of me. When I was given a choice, I took it. Instead of accepting a death sentence, I chose life."

Paul

Effective therapy is about getting past the mind and into the heart. This has been my unwavering philosophy throughout my career as a registered nurse, non-denominational minister and transpersonal hypnotherapist. My hypnosis method can take up to four or five hours in order to establish a solid connection and presence within the deeper levels of consciousness, where we find a fertile environment for life's compass to reset itself and for miracles to manifest through connection with the heart. I work strategically with both sides of the brain—the logical side and the creative side— through an approach tailored to individual needs, marrying the two hemispheres in a very deliberate, creative fashion. Typically, when the client is deeply relaxed and connecting to their body's innate wisdom, they describe sensations within the body that indicate something palpable is happening.

At well over six feet tall with the build of a football linebacker, Paul flew across Canada to have a session with me in Alberta. Upon his arrival, he reported that he was not religious, not spiritual, an atheist, and a disbeliever in life after death. He had been diagnosed with aggressive small cell lung cancer three months prior to his trip to see me. His lymph nodes were involved, and a recent MRI showed lesions in his liver and his brain. Up to this point, he had refused chemotherapy and radiation therapy. I inquired as to why he had chosen to come such a long distance for spiritually-guided therapy. He explained that his colleague, a physician, had come for a session and that he was "a changed man." He said, "I want what he's got."

Once we added a few soft pillows and darkened the room, Paul slid smoothly into a deep trance. I anticipated the usual session: a few questions answered by intuition, then a few questions followed by a deeper knowing, then a few questions answered by his innate Higher Self. However, for the next two hours and fifteen minutes, not one word was spoken by Paul. His eyelids blinking even though his eyes remained closed, he experienced not one muscle movement other than an occasional smile. He was breathing easily with no signs of distress, so I monitored him closely, remaining silent as Paul continued to glide peacefully into his heightened state of awareness. Toward the two-hour and ten minute mark, his facial expression taking on a serious, stone-like appearance, he quietly but emphatically reported, "We're done."

I counted him out, noticing a smile begin to form from ear to ear. When asked what he had been experiencing for over two hours, he giggled, stating that his time 'away' felt like no more than 10 minutes, during which time he experienced brilliant white light, which he described as moving throughout his body in a wavelike motion, bringing with it warmth to his four extremities and tingling in his hands.

Six weeks later, Paul's MRI was clear.

Ralph

Having been diagnosed with diabetes mellitus Type 2 at the age of 29, Ralph (now 67) had been losing his vision for several years due to diabetic retinopathy. The vision in his left eye was still reasonably good, however his right eye was considered to be legally blind. His blood glucose readings were labile, and he struggled with constant neuropathic pain in his right lower leg and foot. He came to my Healing Room from the west coast of Canada, accompanied by his adult son who was the designated driver.

Over the past year, Ralph had been having many dreams in which he was an eagle flying just a few feet above the ground, searching for prey. The dreams were in color; however, the colors were what Ralph described as 'dull and muddy.' Having guided him to wherever his Higher Self wanted him to find the seed of the problem, he was taken back to a past life as a warrior in ancient Greece. During his time at war, his wife, whom he adored, left him for another man. His last thought in that lifetime was that he would never 'see' love again. He believed that he had given so much in his relationship with his wife, that he would never offer the 'sweetness of love' to another woman. The despair he felt was so deeply embedded within his soul's memory that he carried it into this lifetime. Through his transpersonal hypnotherapy session, he offered forgiveness and he invited healing.

In an email about two weeks after his session, he reported that at one point during his journey back to the coast, he felt an overwhelming desire to close his functioning eye. He was shocked. He could read the road signs and billboards without difficulty, leading him to cry uncontrollably. He reported a feeling of increased warmth in his affected eye for the next half hour.

Upon returning to his home, Ralph's wife did not believe that his vision could be restored through hypnosis and he eventually succumbed to her frequent statements of disbelief. Over the following six months, Ralph's vision deteriorated considerably at which time he opted to return for a second hypnotherapy session. Upon his return, we clearly established his own role in setting personal boundaries against the disbelief of others. We discussed how the body tells us something is amiss through symptoms and that his thoughts, feelings, emotions, and beliefs impact his health in untold ways. Once he learned to accept his own power in the healing process, the vision in his affected eye returned once again.

After four years, Ralph's vision remains normal. His blood glucose levels have been more stable and he experiences only occasional discomfort in his right outer foot. He reports being able to 'see' the error of his ways in allowing his wife's limited beliefs to override his own, thereby impacting his ability to heal himself.

Betty

Betty, 79, was a long-term care resident. I was the hospice RN assigned to oversee her end-of-life care and assist the nursing staff to provide appropriate hospice-focused care by routinely visiting her at the facility. Betty had been struggling with cardiomyopathy for several years. She had been my patient for nearly a year during which time we grew quite fond of one another, often sharing jokes and stories of our childhoods. When I visited her on a particular Wednesday, she announced that she would be "dying on Friday." She described having been visited the previous night by angels who told her she would be reunited with her long-deceased husband. Their cryptic message to Betty was, "It's time to gather the daisies." I asked if there was anything I could do for her as she prepared for her final journey. I explained that I would be out of town on the weekend but that the on-call RN from hospice would be available if she should need anything at all.

She then asked if it would be appropriate to visit me the way the angels had visited her. I said that I would welcome a visit, wished her a smooth journey and offered her a warm hug, knowing that I may not see Betty in person again.

On Friday night, I felt a gentle pressure on my left arm. I was alone at the time and I recall how vividly it felt as though my arm were being massaged. Startled by a sound downstairs, I left the bedroom to investigate, only to find that the vase of daisies in the living room was tipped over in the middle of the floor, several feet from the table upon which it had been centered.

The following Monday morning I received a call from the

hospice RN who had been on duty over the weekend, indicating that Betty passed away at 10:30 on Friday evening. She closed her eyes for the last time, after having been assisted to bed by a health care aide who was working her first shift at the facility. The new employee's name was Daisy.

Jean

Jean was 81, unable to speak, feed herself or hold her head up on her own when she succumbed to a four-year decline with progressive supra-nuclear palsy, a neurological disease with symptoms similar to those of Parkinson's disease. A deeply spiritual woman, Jean read the Bible every night before bed, counting her blessings and asking for further guidance from her Creator. She knew the words to many spiritual songs, and her favorite hymn was 'How Great Thou Art.' She always said she would come back with "a report from the other side" if she was the first one to die. My last words to her were a whisper encouraging her to go to the Light and also to remind her to send a report from the other side. Jean was also my mother.

Jean died on December 12, 2011. Eight days later, I was at my desk at work when I received a phone call from my sister, Judi, who was at the house while the piano tuner was occupied downstairs in the family room. After suggesting that I sit down first, she described how the piano tuner had spent the morning plunking away at the keyboard, one note after another, as she worked at her computer, upstairs. After a brief moment of quiet, he began playing a sweeping rendition of 'How Great Thou Art.' When Judi went downstairs to tell him how lovely it sounded, he confessed that he rarely played hymns, but he felt deeply inspired to play that particular piece. Then, a mere two or three minutes later, my sister received a phone call from the funeral home advising that our mother's ashes were ready to be picked up. Later that night, Judi was wakened by feeling a hand on her shoulder. It was firm yet it offered a sense of comfort and calm. She instinctively felt Mom was letting her know 'all is well.'

Then, on a cold winter night in January of 2020, it was my turn. Although I slept well that night, just before sunrise, I felt three sharp pokes on my shoulder, and I heard Mom's voice call my name from the other side of the room. It was so clear that I sat bolt upright, answering her call.

Over the years, my mother has fulfilled her promise to connect in gentle, soothing ways. Although I cannot touch her, I do feel her, and with that comes great comfort, knowing that she remains as close as ever.

Miracles abound…like angels and spirit guides, they are all around us…if only we watch for them and allow their messages to enter our hearts, without expectations, without judgement. Only then will the beauty and rewards of those miracles touch us in very personal ways. We manifest through our beliefs and what we believe creates the life we experience. Choose to experience miracles. Allow them to come into your life and prepare to be pleasantly surprised.

About the Author

Heather Gunn, PhD(C), MSN, RN (retired), CCHt

A registered nurse from 1979 to 2019 in Canada and the U.S., Heather is also a non-denominational minister, nursing educator, and master transpersonal clinical hypnotherapist, currently completing a PhD in Integrative Medicine. After experiencing the power of the quantum field during a near death experience, she studied Reiki, becoming a Reiki master teacher over 30 years ago.

Through the years, Heather witnessed the depth of beauty within the spiritual dimension while working with her patients, finding that we learn so much about living from those who are dying. Their messages confirm that we are in control of our health and wellbeing by bringing the human spirit into the healing process. Her clients' spiritual and cultural backgrounds vary from Mormon, Muslim, Mennonite and Hutterite to Buddhist, Baptist, agnostic, and atheist. Her clients have ranged in age from 6 to 89, coming from Canada, the U.S., and across the globe. They struggle with health challenges ranging from anxiety, depression, and gender identity concerns to MS, Parkinson's disease, and cancer. One Spirit Integrative Medicine is situated on six acres of gentle, rolling hills at the foothills of the Alberta Rockies, along with three miniature donkeys to keep an eye on the coyotes and other indigenous critters.

Contact Information:

One Spirit Integrative Medicine
Fort Macleod, Alberta, Canada
Cell: 403-894-2622
Website: www.onespirit.ca
Email: onespiritall@gmail.com
YouTube: QHHT Regression Hypnosis – The Truth Be Told

A CHALLENGE TO TRUTH

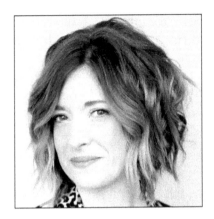

Cari Rosno

April 2013 provided a poignant moment in American history, a moment where the foundation of the safety of a country was yet again brought into question. A day of celebration turned tragic. For me this was a day that shook me to the depths of my soul leaving me nowhere to go but inward.

I had picked up running in 2009 after the birth of our third child as a way to release stress from a life that had me moving in all sorts of directions. I was a mother of three children, wife, business owner, board member, and liaison to small businesses and host home for a house-based church. Running was my time to escape and I was good at it. Running in only my second marathon, without a goal in mind, I qualified to run the Boston marathon. Truly a marathoner's dream… a dream, which in a moment, I picked up and made mine.

I love the city of Boston on Patriots' Day. The weather turns toward spring, the people are festive, and the city welcoming and warm to all whom have traveled in. The morning of April 15th, 2013 had an air of celebration. The excitement was palpable as I made my way that morning to the buses transporting us to the start of the marathon. The weather was cool but comfortable and perfect for running. I remember thinking, I've made it!

The beginning of the race was amazing. I was on pace to match my time for qualifying and I felt like I was floating on air. Around mile 15 things turned and my body started to get heavy, my muscles cramped, and my pace slowed drastically. As I worked my way through the city for the remaining miles, I made an agreement with myself, the same agreement I had made before, just finish the race and then I'll immediately go to the medical tent.

Without surprise, but with intense pain, I crossed the finish line soaking up all the cheers as my last bit of energy propelled me forward and I found my way into the welcoming arms of the volunteers and nurses.

I couldn't have been there long, perhaps 20 minutes by the time I was checked in, attended to and awaiting further assistance, when it happened. It happened in a wave of events that will never leave my mind. An explosive sound that hit the air like a wave, causing all to pause and look at one another in curiosity. Then it happened again, though this time it was undeniable. In a moment, a flash of a second that literally both shook the earth and made the world stand still, we knew. It was a bomb... bombs had just been set off.

In this moment, terror not only tore through the heart of the city, it tore through me as well. That day's events were indescribable, confusing, shocking. The next day proved to be no different as my husband, mother and I walked in a state of disbelief through a city that was in the heat of a manhunt. The streets were lined with military personnel and media from across the country. As we stood looking down the desolate war torn street, me wearing my official 2013 Boston Marathon jacket, a reporter politely tapped me on the shoulder asking about my experience running Boston. I said nothing, turned and walked away with a voice in my head saying, "It is not my story to tell." This was a denial of my own truth, which would prove devastating in the months and years to come.

Within a matter of weeks I went from running marathons to being unable to walk up a flight of stairs unassisted. I became bedridden and had glimpses of hopelessness as illness ravaged my body. Over the course of the next three years I would slowly uncover diagnoses through a journey that had to begin with learning to trust myself: chronic Lyme disease, Hashimoto's, Epstein-Barr, heavy metal toxicities and multiple autoimmune conditions just to name a few. This is where my challenge to find truth begins.

In 2016 I was referred to a healer who guided me to address the source of my illnesses—my mind. Yeah, you heard me right, my beliefs and thoughts needed healing alongside my body. I, like everyone else, have lived a life. A life with people involved and feelings, where experiences happen, death occurs, and love is misinterpreted. I needed to sit with all of it. I had been holding onto emotions and anger that I thought, as many of my clients do, I had worked through. I had talked about the death of our stillborn daughter and had seen a marriage counselor. I had discussed things with my parents and addressed my broken heart. I had talked and recounted and relived until I was done reliving, done talking about it, yet I knew I still had "stuff" that needed moved.

I was challenged to dig deep into myself, to sit in the pain without distraction and address limiting beliefs that played out in my life. As I peeled back the layers of trauma and shifted my perspective, healing came. I released anger and outdated thoughts that I was unaware were directing me. When I did this and found true love for myself, let go of fear and started honoring myself above all…everything healed. Years of insomnia were gone overnight. Over the course of a year I overcame it all and completely changed my life in the most spectacular of ways. My relationships became so much more fulfilling, I sold the marketing company I owned, and I became the person I always knew I could and wanted to be. I began living my truth instead of everyone else's.

I had never experienced anything so profound that touched every aspect of my life in such beautiful ways. I have always known the power of words, but I had no idea the power of my thoughts and how shifting the way I perceived the world could put me in the driver's seat of my own life. No longer was I a passenger waiting for the next thing, I create every step. Having seen what

I am capable of and understanding how to walk alongside others in their journey, I had to step up to inspire and guide.

My healing is just one of the many miracles I have had the opportunity to witness. Working with clients I am constantly in awe as to the power of the mind, the power of words and how in any given moment we have the opportunity to change. We all have the power to experience these miracles… now I simply teach people how.

Nick is a client that I had the privilege to witness find his truth, change his mind and create a new reality. He is 13 and a boy who loves sports but unfortunately had come down hard while snowboarding, hit his head and suffered a concussion. He was missing school, unable to play sports, watch TV, read, or engage in anything stimulating. After three weeks of doctor visits, he fell ill with something similar to the 24-hour flu and began having trouble sleeping. He could fall asleep, but within hours would wake and be up for the remainder of the night. A week and a half into this his mother brought him to see me. When Nick arrived, I spoke with him and his mom about his prognosis.

"We went to see the doctor and he said, 'Normal adults and a small percentage of teens will heal within 30 days.' He continued, "I am not one of those and have two to three more weeks of healing," Nick proclaimed.

"Your mom mentioned you have also been having a hard time sleeping, maybe nightmares? Is that correct?" I asked Nick.

"Yep, I have the same dream." He says as he begins to get visibly upset. "I am in a black box and they keep taking everything I love away from me. My toys, my dog, my parents and my papa."

Nick and I began working together and as I helped him addresswhat was happening in his subconscious mind through a form of meditation, he began unraveling the dream. It was one in which he felt like he was being punished and that he would lose everything. As we shifted memories and situations that he had experienced, the dream changed as well.

"Nick, you know you can change your mind, right? Can we have God teach you that you are normal and that you can decide when you want to get better? Can God show you that you can be better now if you want?" I asked.

"Yes."

Through meditation, intention and connection with the energy of creation we shifted his perspective and subconscious programming. When our one session together came to a close, Nick had a huge smile on his face visibly showing he felt better. We hugged and he hurried off. That evening, Nick went to dinner with his parents and attended a semi-pro hockey game, all without any discomfort. As the night ended, he went home and ran up to bed, hopped in, and fell fast asleep. Nick simply changed his mind. His concussion completely healed, and Nick immediately received clearance to go back to snowboarding and playing soccer.

How does that happen? How did he shift so quickly and have the ability to experience such a miracle, an instant healing? We worked together to understand what his mind was doing, how his subconscious was protecting him and where the source of the pain was. Once the limiting belief was located, we worked with the energy of creation to change it, rewire his brain and shift the subconscious process into something that can now serve him better.

Nick's story is amazing! The ability to heal ourselves is miraculous and innate in whom we are. Now what if we could go a step further—what if—you could heal yourself, your children, your families and your ancestors all at the same time? Hear me out on this. I am going to share a story that gives a glimpse of that possibility.

Shadow had come into my family as a very young puppy during a time when our elder dog Sadie seemed to be within her last months of life and my middle son was struggling with severe anxiety and depression. He needed a buddy and Shadow somehow fell into our laps. He was instantly welcomed and brought nurturing and love like we had never experienced. He was a spark of PURE LOVE.

Shadow was a healer in his own right, giving a growly voice to pain and snuggling close. He was always at my side during meditation, healing and brought smiles to clients immediately upon their arrival. Taking walks was the special time that Shadow and I shared away from everyone, just the two of us. He loved his walks.

Shadow was all smiles as we took a walk on our annual

camping trip in late June, a walk he had waited for. He was an expressive dog and while I knew he was happy I also knew he was ready to turn back. We sat in the shade for a while and rested before turning to return to the campsite. As we walked back, I noticed that Shadow seemed to be panting a little heavier than normal and he rested a little more, however between stops he was all energy, always running to the next shady tree. The last five minutes seemed to take forever, his back legs started to give out periodically, but as usual he would bounce up and run. We finished our walk and Shadow immediately crawled to the cool concrete under our camper.

I checked on him often and through his smile and softer breathing I suspected all to have calmed. I returned to my conversation with friends. Moments later I again looked over to check on him and found my daughter's friend standing over him with her dad and knew by the look on their faces that all was not well. I ran to where they were with visible concern—and I simply got *the look* and a head shake, *no*. Chaos ensued. He was gone. I don't recall all the details of the next moments; I was in a shocked grief and despair of "What did I do? How could I have let him overheat? How could I have done this?" I collapsed in the grass behind the camper and stayed there, comforted by those closest to me as they held space for my pain. They were a shoulder to lean on, a liaison in conversation with my husband who had traveled two hours away to pick up our daughter, and the adult chaperoning my two older boys from the marina on the river 30 minutes away.

When we went home, I couldn't face them. I couldn't talk to my boys or even walk into our house. I was riddled with grief and overwhelmed by guilt. I needed clarity, a different perspective, and understanding of what had happened. I have learned and know that I can find the answers I am longing for in meditation and with the energy of creation. That evening as I submerged myself in the bath to connect with something greater than myself, I felt compelled to find truth.

I lit a candle, added some salts and a little essential oil, allowing my tears to stir with the water. I asked Creator to show me what had happened and to provide clarity to the situation and to any beliefs that had arisen during the day. Immediately upon stepping into a meditative state, allowing my mind to quiet and opening my thoughts, a space created through desperation, I received the following:

"He had an enlarged heart. It was his time; he chose the time. He didn't want you near, he knew you would do anything to save him, and he didn't want the kids around. It was his decision, he wanted that last walk with you," said Creator.

"Can you release the trauma? Do I resent myself and do I believe I killed him?" I asked.

"Of course you do, but it was his choice," replied the same loving voice.

"Can we change the way I am seeing this?" I inquired.

"Of course you can. You do realize this started yesterday?" At this point I was taken to memories of the day before where Shadow was whining for what seemed to be no reason, sitting in the backseat of the car and later lounging under a shade tree. This realization was profound and provided an incredible healing opportunity for me to see the events from a different perspective. After roughly 30 minutes I resurfaced from the bath and was in a better space, a place of love and calm, able to support the rest of my family, as I desired to.

Then the most incredible thing happened. Later that night my middle son came to join me in bed and curling up right next to me he said, "Mom, I wanted to be mad at you all day today. I wanted to be mad at you for taking Shadow for a walk. But it wasn't your fault, you didn't do anything wrong. I actually think this started yesterday. You know how Sadie always licks you? Shadow never did, but he did yesterday, and I think that was him trying to tell me goodbye."

My moment of clarity in shifting my perspective and healing my mind had provided a healing that transcended time and space. It healed my son in the moment it healed me. In honoring ourselves, we honor our experiences and our pain. We open ourselves to forgiveness, love and a deeper understanding of the amazing creators that we are. We are infinitely powerful. Through the power of meditation, intention and shifting the mind, healing occurs. It penetrates spiritually, mentally and physically healing the generations.

How will you find your truth?

About the Author

Cari Rosno

Cari is a global manifestation coach and healing instructor on a journey to challenge truth. Her personal journey of overcoming PTSD, chronic Lyme disease, Hashimoto's thyroiditis, and other health complications has equipped her to teach others how to release their own trauma and awaken to their true potential. Cari offers workshops and retreats, personal coaching, and digital tools to help individuals own their power and take responsibility for creating the life they desire.

Learn more at www.carirosno.com.

WHERE MIRACLES COME FROM

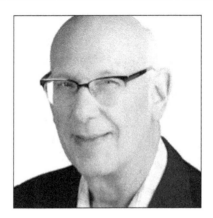

Dr. Dennis Permann

I have a different perspective from most healers. Oh, I'm clear that healing is an inside-out phenomenon, and I know that the miracles that patients report are due to their natural inherent recuperative ability. That is part of the miracle; the patient comes to our offices with the doctor already inside. We facilitate the process by eliminating stress and friction in the system, and the person heals organically.

The reason my viewpoint varies from a typical practitioner is that I retired from active patient care 32 years ago, opting instead to serve the profession by guiding doctors toward best-in-class protocols and identity-based personal and professional growth. Ten thousand clients later, I've developed a special appreciation for the miracles that manifest in chiropractic offices worldwide.

Most of the miracles I get to participate in these days are miracles of individual breakthrough—doctors who were floundering in practice who discover their greatness and created the practices and lifestyles of their dreams, as well as already successful doctors who blaze new trails to ultra-prosperity.

These personal triumphs each represent hundreds or thousands of patients and dozens or hundreds of miracles. That was why I moved from practice into coaching, I wanted a bigger game.

Yet, I have many wonderful memories of patients who had miraculous responses under my care. Please let me share a few of my favorites.

It was a typical Saturday night about five years ago, and my lovely wife Regina and I decided to hit a new Japanese restaurant in town. We headed over with the best of intentions, but when we arrived, it was closed. How odd for a new restaurant to be closed on a Saturday night, but hey, there are so many places to eat in Huntington, it wasn't a problem, and we headed to a familiar dining establishment.

We were seated and handed menus, and while we were deciding what to eat, I got the unmistakable feeling that someone was eyeballing me. I glanced up from my menu and a guy at the next table was full on staring at me.

I smiled and tried to redirect my attention back to selecting my meal, but he was still eyeballing me, so I looked right at him.

"Are you Dr. Dennis?" he asked.

"Well, yes," I answered. "Do I know you?"

"You don't recognize me," he said.

"You know, I meet a lot of people. Where would I know you from?"

He leaned back so I could see his wife sitting next to him, smiling. "You don't remember her?"

And then it came to me. These nice people were two of my very last new patients before I sold my practice to go into full-time teaching and coaching. They came to me because they were having fertility issues, unable to conceive, and were told that I had great results with such patients. On my way out of practice, I had heard that they were expecting, but I never did connect with them after I left.

As recognition dawned on me, the guy pointed at me, and then pointed at the handsome, dark-haired young man seated across from him and his wife, and proclaimed in a loud, clear voice, "YOU... are responsible... for HIM!"

My wife dropped the menu with a horrified look on her

face. While the people at the adjacent tables tittered amongst themselves with knowing winks and nods, I quickly filled Regina in, and we all had a good chuckle and a joyful exchange. After 27 years of parenthood, they finally got to close the loop and say thank you for the miracle of their son's birth, serendipitously sitting next to us at a restaurant we almost didn't go to.

One of the reasons I attracted difficult and unusual cases is because of the specialty work that I learned and applied. A typical day might include patients with severe neurological disease, young families coming for wellness care, people with an assortment of aches and pains, and of course the patients who had been everywhere and defaulted to a chiropractor as their last resort—how many times have I heard that? This was all before they stopped trying because they were told nothing could be done and they should go home and live with it.

These were the patients I welcomed into my practice, because after all the outside-in practitioners threw up their hands, I knew every patient had something inside that wanted to express itself. It was up to me to clear away anything preventing that. The solution invariably came from addressing their physical stresses, chemical stresses, emotional stresses, and vibrational stresses. I knew it was my job to see which stresses could be reduced or eliminated, and which stresses needed to be coped with or adapted to, so I could develop my game plan to help them move toward wellness.

Getting their brain healthy was paramount, since a healthy brain is a necessary precondition for all healing. The reason I saw so many miracles even over my short 10 years of practice was because I considered each of these types of disruption in the body's rhythm and function, which set the stage for the patient to respond rapidly and thoroughly.

There was a chiropractor in my area whose father had serious vascular disease. He had already been to the surgeon to have one of his carotid arteries stripped out because it was severely occluded, and his brain suffered from reduced blood flow. They couldn't do both sides at once, of course, because then the brain would get no blood at all. He was scheduled for a second surgery six weeks later, but he was so miserable after that first invasive procedure that he begged his son to find a more natural alternative, so they turned to me.

I knew I had to act quickly, as the surgical date was fast approaching. I scheduled Mr. M for a series of specific adjustments, during which I focused on his circulatory system, his heart, and the relevant neurology, including his vagus nerve. I also used the harmonic vascular enhancement technique I learned from M.L. Rees, applying specially programmed crystals to balance the energy of his blood vessels. This may sound flaky, but healing is microscopic and influenced by subtle forces. It's not weird that crystals are used in computers, radios, cell phones and watches, so why not healing? I saw incredible changes in people when I was able to tune their vibration, so they experienced a sense of personal harmony that invariably led to healing and wellness.

So, I began Mr. M's care, and he started to improve—dizziness receded, fewer headaches and then none, more vitality. And then, the moment of truth. He went in for his examination before surgery, to find out the verdict. His surgeon came out of the testing room sputtering, "How is it possible? The second vessel was clearer than the first! It must have been a misdiagnosis, there's no other explanation."

Mr. M just smiled. He couldn't tell the surgeon why he was able to avoid the second surgery because his doctor would never believe it anyway. But this miracle saved him from that painful invasive procedure, extending his life significantly.

I will leave you with one more example. This is a story of the miracle that got away.

I remember when Jeff first came to my office. He was 19 years old, three years after a diving accident left him a quadriplegic, paralyzed from the neck down. He was a smiley kid, who faced his disability with determination and a sense of humor. I instantly liked him, and I appreciated his willingness to do whatever it takes to get better. Not that it wasn't an ordeal for him to come to my office. His attendant, a burly fellow named Mack who looked over Jeff like a mama hen, was careful to help me every step of the way, getting him out of the wheelchair and onto the adjusting table, watching closely as I adjusted Jeff's skull, his spine, his extremities, his organs, balanced his energy. Everywhere I looked, there were issues that needed attention, and I concentrated all of my expertise to see if I could give this terrific young man a bit of his life back.

Well, wouldn't you know it, he began to respond—not by getting up and dancing, but little things: starting to perspire in areas that previously were completely dry, shrugging his shoulders a little, and he even reported that his male functions were beginning to return. We were elated that his body had some ability to heal, and we all felt good about the progress.

Then one day, after a particularly complex adjustment, Mack pulled me aside and asked an honest question. "Doc, what do you think are the chances that Jeff will walk again?"

I was in full doctor mode, and I remember my response like it was yesterday. "Well, you know, he had a very severe injury to his neck and brain, and we have to be reasonable in our expectations..." As the words came out, I would have given anything to be able to run after them and shove them back in my mouth. His face darkened, and I knew I had screwed up really bad.

I never saw Jeff again. I had committed the worst mistake any miracle worker can ever make, a cardinal error of professional immaturity—I denied my patient hope.

Hope is the missing link that connects healers with miracles. Hope generates an energy field of its own, so the patient gets the most out of any intervention, out of all proportion to what might be anticipated. Hope turns on the next level of metabolism and repair, going beyond the mechanical to invoke the higher powers. Hope is the contrast between a patient feeling relief and a patient experiencing the miraculous healing and wellness benefits for which chiropractic is famous. Hope is the difference that makes the difference.

When I played it safe and covered my tracks, I shut down the whole miracle process with my ignorance and clumsiness. Many times after that, I wondered what might have happened in Jeff's life if I only showed up bigger at that crossroads. I pray that Jeff made it into another chiropractor's office and made the shifts and improvement that led to his best possible outcomes, in spite of my own failure. I know his resiliency meant anything was possible, and if it was his destiny to walk, perhaps he found a healer who got out of the way and let the miracle occur.

There is a natural rightness to what we do, a consistency with universal law that gives us massive power we must engage with extraordinary humility. You see, if you believe that it's you doing the miracles, and then you must accept responsibility when they do not happen.

Rather, the miracles come from a place some might call spiritual, others might call esoteric or quantum, but whatever you call it, it is not so much under our control as it is available for our appreciation. Chiropractic philosophers refer to this as the Innate Principle, the inborn ability we all carry with us, the intelligence and wisdom of the body and mind that regulates physiology and restores function whenever it is distorted. All healing comes from within; even when there is a successful intervention, like an adjustment, medication, or surgery, still the healing always comes from within.

So then, miracles are natural occurrences, setting the wheels in motion with our loving care triggers the miracle; it doesn't cause it.

And that is good news indeed—it explains why there are miracles occurring daily in chiropractic and wellness offices worldwide, under the guidance of masters and novices; chiropractors, osteopaths, MDs and lay healers; specialists and general practitioners, from every school, style, technique, and every personality type. The common factor? The patient's ability to respond. Innate intelligence synthesizes the raw materials into miracles. It is the patient's inborn power, the skill and expertise you apply as the operator, and whatever confluence of conditions are required to make the magic happen.

When I was finishing my second year of Chiropractic College, I bought my first adjusting table in 1978, an orange Naugahyde bench with woodgrain Formica and the fittings that I needed for my particular approach. I had just gotten it home when Regina's friend and co-worker Suzy called, saying she was bent over in pain, asking if there was anything I could do to help.

Well, brave and stupid is not usually a great combination, but I said, "Of course, come on over and let's see what we can do."

When she hobbled into my den, I got a bit of a chill. This was my first real patient, and I had no license, no insurance, no experience, no x-rays, and only enough knowledge to get myself in trouble. But I knew she needed me, so I threw caution to the wind and trusted that I would figure it out.

I sat her on my orange Naugahyde table, palpated her neck, and I could feel the top bone (the atlas) sticking way out to the right. I laid her down on the table with her right side up so I could take a contact on that bone, and I prepared to make the adjustment. I squared my shoulders to the table, placed Nail Point One on the offending vertebra, and reinforced my contact by rolling my indifferent pisiform into the anatomical snuffbox. I positioned my episternal notch directly above the contact point and began to breathe with the patient. At the exact right moment, I flicked my elbows, thrusting smoothly downward with a slight rotational torque, setting that misaligned bone into motion so the body could put it where it belonged.

After all, I don't know where that bone should be... but the body does. So confidently and resourcefully, I delivered that adjustment with positive expectancy and faith that it was naturally right, and that innate intelligence would know precisely what to do with my loving concussion of forces. So I had just given that adjustment to my very first patient. There she was, lying on her side after I did what I was going to do, one bone, one thrust. Now what?

I asked her to stay there until the pulsing in her neck stopped, and the musculature felt supple, and then I brought her up into a sitting position. The look on Suzy's face was priceless. She started scanning the room, as if to say, "Didn't I have pain when I came in here? What happened to my pain?" I had participated in my very first chiropractic miracle, where a patient went from antalgic agony to feeling fine in minutes.

One last word to the wise. We love the drama of someone getting instant relief from our care, and it is intoxicating. But we must remember, it is no less miraculous to offer a right adjustment to a well person. The work of innate intelligence is just as important in a healthy person as it is in a sick person. So, remember to share your miracles with those who are symptomatic and those who are not. Everyone deserves to enjoy the miraculous healing and wellness benefits for which chiropractic is famous.

About the Author

Dr. Dennis Permann, DC

Dennis Perman, DC, award-winning author, speaker, healer and coach, has trained thousands of Doctors of Chiropractic, wellness professionals and paraprofessionals over three decades. Co-Founder of The Masters Circle Global, he has delivered hundreds of presentations to enthusiastic audiences throughout North America and Europe.

In six books, hundreds of newsletters, over a thousand online columns and dozens of audio and video products, Dr. Perman offers his original materials and perspectives on self-development, communication, leadership, health, business, team-building, personality engineering, and brain-based wellness. His innovative Capacity Technology™ provides a roadmap to personal growth and professional fulfillment.

Dennis is the executive producer of TMCtv, the world's largest online video success library for chiropractors, with over 500 hours of programming featuring 125 speakers. He co-produced the monthly audio-magazine MasterTalk for 14 years, interviewed over 150 celebrities, and has published his free e-column, "Message of the Week" since September 1997, over 1,100 editions, and more than half a million words.

For information on speaking or coaching or to subscribe to the "Message of the Week," please contact dennis@themasterscircle.net or call 800-451-4514.

THE ABSENCE OF A MIRACLE...

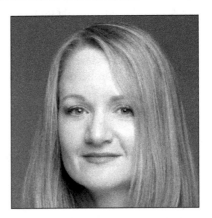

Dr. Katinka van der Merwe

Most doctors were called into healing by a moment, a miracle, a lightning rod. This moment was usually the birth of a great desire to help those who are suffering, to embrace the sick and broken, to make this world a better place. The first 34 years of my life, I was missing my moment. As the daughter of a great chiropractor known for helping the hopeless, I was born into a life that was all I knew. My choices, I thought, were shaped by my desire to please my dad, to make him proud of me, and to live up to his expectations. I had no great reason to become a healer, other than wanting to follow in my father's footsteps. I was missing the "why."

After graduation in Dallas in 2000, I joined my newly immigrated family in the beautiful Fayetteville, Arkansas. My dad had recently set out in practice on his own again. My family was full of hardworking people, shaped by forefathers familiar with being adrift on a strange continent, and carving out a new way of life. I spent the first eight years of my career steeped in misery, knowing that I lacked passion, that I was a going through the motions, an imposter. I did not love my work and knew that I was merely surviving professionally. I was missing the magic that breathes fire into every fulfilling career. Nevertheless, I labored on. My family was embraced by the tight knit community hugged by green hills and lakes, where people still brought you fresh vegetables from their gardens, and everyone knew most everyone else. I questioned my life's choices. Saddled by crippling student loans and my dad's pride in working next to me, I carried on.

One Saturday, 11 years ago, I received a fateful phone call. "Can you come to the hospital? Tommy was hurt. It is bad." Tommy van Zandt was an ex-Texan, a successful local commercial realtor, a businessman, and a family man of two teenage boys and lovely wife—both patients of mine. Tommy was in the prime of his life. He was handsome, charismatic, and beloved by our community. That morning, Tommy had climbed up a 16-foot ladder in his backyard to cut down a branch off of a tree that had been killed by a crippling ice storm our area had recently suffered. The branch came loose, knocking Tommy off the ladder onto his back.

The fall had crushed Tommy's cervical spine, leaving him unable to breathe. Robyn, his wife, had found him in the nick of time, able to call 911 and save his life. Tommy was put in ICU here in Fayetteville. Tommy's family was scared and desperate. They had hope that somehow, alternative care would succeed where allopathic medicine had reached its limits. At the time, the neurosurgeon that was treating Tommy was a patient of my dad, and I was allowed to go treat him in ICU.

It was a sunny afternoon when I found myself standing next to Tommy's bed, surrounded by his family. This strong, dynamic human being was hooked up to breathing equipment and sedated. I looked at that beautiful family surrounding me, hoping that somehow, I could provide the miracle they were aching for. I have never in my unsatisfying career thus far felt more powerless, more impotent, more hopeless. The miracle I would have loved to give Tommy did not come through me that day. I left the hospital, made it to my car and cried like a baby. I cried for my helplessness and I cried because not so deep down, I felt incompetent and powerless.

I would go on and treat Tommy for months afterward. I

treated him at Craig Rehab in Denver and eventually at home. He would require a team of caregivers from thereon out. He had lost the ability to walk, move from the head down, feed himself, and breathe on his own. His injury was catastrophic and life altering, the stuff of which nightmares are made.

You may ask yourself, in a book of miracles, what this story has to contribute. You see, miracles, I have learned, are not always instant moments, magically giving us the outcomes we long for from the depths of our souls. Miracles may take weeks, months, or years. Miracles may be formed purposely by our hard work and the decision and determination to change. They may be born in the moment when we hit rock bottom. Tommy was my rock bottom. Up until Tommy, I was just going through the motions in my career. I believed I lacked that X-factor that turned ordinary doctors into great healers. Tommy was my watershed moment. I could have given up, but somehow, that experience became the spark that lit my passion.

I understood that the human body had limits, and sometimes, even the best healers could not overcome physical limitations. Sometimes, the body is just too broken to fix. More often than not though, there is hope. I understood this philosophy. My very upbringing had trained me to believe in the body's miraculous, innate ability to heal itself. However, I had not allowed myself to learn as much as I could. There were techniques, technologies, and methods in the world that I had not examined. I was operating below my full potential while I was surrounded by tens of thousands of Tommies and untold suffering while I denied, questioned, and forgot my calling to heal the broken and suffering.

I changed and became obsessed with opening my heart and mind to learning. I made a deal with the Universe that if knowledge was sent to me, I would open myself to learning and serving. I spent weekends traveling every corner of the world, learning from those treating some of the most helpless cases across the globe. I vowed that when my next Tommy came, I would be ready. I was thirsty for knowledge and open to learning. I found mentors who believed in me and who were willing to guide me. I knew my moment would come, that something great would happen. The seed had been sown and it was being fertilized. I waited for what would grow.

One ordinary Tuesday in practice, I met Carlos. He suffered from Complex Regional Pain Syndrome (CRPS), a nervous system disorder of unknown origin. CRPS is a condition that starts after a seemingly innocent enough injury, such as (even simple) surgeries, fractures, or something as simple as a needle stick. CRPS causes immeasurable, devastating pain. Patients describe the pain associated with CRPS as worse than childbirth. As if that is not bad enough, CRPS may spread, eventually consuming the body inside and out. There is no medical cure for CRPS. It is known as one of the "suicide diseases," and for good reason. The first thing a newly diagnosed patient typically does upon receiving a diagnosis is research this condition on the internet, only to discover that there is no cure, no way out of the daily hell of burning pain. Eventually, it often breaks the spirit of even the most courageous of patients. Death may seem like the only way out for many.

Traditionally, CRPS is managed through nerve blocks, ketamine treatments (a strong tranquilizer used for animals such as horses), opioids, Fentanyl patches and spinal cord stimulators implanted next to the spinal cord. In Carlos's case, it had progressed and attacked his gastrointestinal tract, causing burning pain every time he tried to eat. When I met Carlos, he was forced to give up his career as a police officer because of his illness. He had lost 60 pounds and his pain was out of any medical control. He had gone through all the standard treatments for CRPS, all providing no real relief.

Carlos was accompanied by his wife that day, holding their nine-month old baby boy, Sean. Carlos was in severe pain, his head down and skin drained of all color. The whole time I was taking his medical history, his wife was his voice. Carlos was sitting with his head down, in too much pain to speak. He had been in countless medical offices before. To him, I was just the next in a long line of doctors who could not help him and did not understand. His wife, Tonya, told me that she feared for his life. Carlos had lost the will to live. Carlos that day reminded me of one of my favorite poems by William Yeats, "Sailing to Byzantium." It goes: "An aged man is but a paltry thing, a tattered coat upon a stick, unless soul clap its hands and sing." Carlos had ceased to live, although he was alive.

Carlos's wife, however, was not ready to let him go. She had begged him to try one more time, to not give up, to fight for their son. Carlos just wanted the pain to stop. Any other aspiration and ambition no longer mattered. He had gone from living to surviving poorly, minute by minute. He had exhausted his medical options. I carefully took down his medical history. The whole time I thought, "This is it. This is it! This is the kind of misery I was born to relieve." Finally, Carlos looked up, directly into my eyes. His face was haunted. "I don't believe you can help me. I am here for my wife." His words were honest and direct.

My heart stopped. What if I could not help him? I stepped into our break room, doubt coursing through me. I had been preparing for this moment, and now I was petrified. My dad happened to be there. As always, I turned to him for advice. "What if I can't help this man?" His reply was simple: "What if you can?"

I treated Carlos that day with a simple technique designed to improve vagus nerve function. Logically, I thought that it was a good fit for his condition. If the vagus nerve was once again communicating, it could, in theory, decrease his inflammation and therefore decrease his pain. However, I had no idea if it would work. My efforts seemed too small to make a dent in his misery. Carlos left; his pain decreased. He went to a restaurant and ate a full meal, causing him no pain. The next day, he returned, his color improved, and his pain dramatically decreased. On Carlos's face I saw the birth of hope. I have since learned that hope is the most powerful ingredient in any healing process. The moment you restore hope, all else becomes possible. I had gained his trust.

Carlos completed his treatment 12 weeks later, all his pain gone. He was a different human being than the one who first walked into my office. I was addicted. Being part of his miracle was the single most thrilling moment of my life. I had found my calling. I became obsessed with helping those patients who could not find help anywhere else, and I vowed that I would bring my skills to others who suffered. Today, nine years later, Carlos is still in remission. Carlos went on to become a youth minister, helping many others who feel hopeless and who have reached rock bottom. Carlos's family got him back, happy and whole, the man he was supposed to be. His son (now 10) is growing up with a father, his wife with a husband.

Carlos woke something up in my soul. Through him, I had found my purpose and true North. I believed that if I build it, they would come, and come, they did. Patients trickled in at first. We were a small clinic and our voice back then was quiet. Our message, however, was powerful and resonated with patients who have been given up on. Our success stories were accumulated, and word started spreading. It is impossible to measure the value of the lives saved by our system, but what is clear is that the positivity of each recovery circles out and touches the lives of loved ones, friends, and communities.

Each story is unique. There was Romeo, a 12-year-old boy from Australia who begged his mom one night to get their gun and end it all. Today, Romeo is once again a normal 13-year-old boy. There was Victorine, the volleyball player from Belgium, on crutches for five years and unwilling to continue on in pain. Currently, Victorine is once again back on the court, two years CRPS-free. There was Philip, who would recover from CRPS and go on to form The Burning Limb Foundation, a non-profit organization designed to fund care not covered by insurance for others in pain. Every story was unique and remarkable, each patient success a miracle.

Since Carlos, I have treated more than 350 patients who suffer from conditions like CRPS, Ehlers Danlos Syndrome (EDS) and other incurable nerve pain. I grew from a staff of three to a staff of 20; every member of my team plucked from all walks of life (waiters, family members of patients, and ex-car salesmen). My number one criteria when selecting staff was compassion for those who suffer and passion for their work. Everything else can be taught. My team is just as driven as I am, and we are making waves in healthcare, capturing the attention of the media and other doctors from all over the world.

Our formula to reach the suffering is simple: tell our story simply and show our miracles. We post every breakthrough on social media, documenting patient progress from the moment a patient comes through our door in a wheelchair to the moment they can run again without pain. People are resonating with our message of hope. Pain should not simply be managed by chemicals or implanted medical devices. Pain should not be accepted. No one should just be given up on. The body is intelligent and magnificent, often capable of healing the most traumatic of injuries, if given the correct support.

Our patients have now come to us from 52 different countries. Soon, we will run out of space as our waiting list growing. In an effort to accommodate our growth we are designing a small hospital that will be named The Spero Clinic. Spero means hope in Latin. Our motto is also Latin: *"Dum Spiro Spero,"* meaning, "While I breathe, I hope."

I did not give Tommy his miracle; he gave me mine. I have used the heartache and sense of hopelessness born from his case to fuel my passion. The gift of working with something you are passionate about is immeasurable, and I cannot ever thank him enough. As for Tommy, he has touched many lives since his injury. He could have shriveled into a life of disability, and instead, Tommy has thrived and become an inspiration to many. He was featured in a book about his experience, written by his brother in-law. Tommy is again very active in the real estate world, and in an interesting twist of fate, was the realtor who found and sold me the piece of land our hospital will soon be built on. In addition, he has inspired many to go on and thrive, no matter the odds. I am grateful every day that his life touched mine. It has taught me that our greatest sorrows carve the mold by which our greatest miracles are formed into existence.

About the Author

Dr. Katinka van der Merwe, DC

Dr. Katinka van der Merwe grew up in Johannesburg, South Africa as the daughter of a successful chiropractic doctor. She followed in her father's footsteps and graduated from Parker College of Chiropractic in 1999. She has since gained a reputation of taking on hopeless and severe patient cases and has gained international attention due to her unprecedented success rates in these cases. She practices in Fayetteville, AR and is the CEO of The Spero Clinic (www.thesperoclinic.com). In 2018, Dr. Katinka was awarded Global Chiropractor of the Year in Atlanta, Georgia by the Masters Circle Global for her outstanding achievement in her profession.

FAIRYTALE FAITH

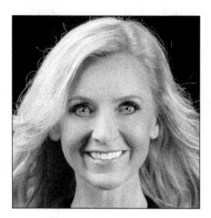

Dr. Carla Burns

"I just opened an email from 23 and Me and it says I have a son... you!"

I will vividly remember this text from my husband for the rest of my life as one of the most incredible manifestations of a miracle I have personally witnessed. Have you seen the movie *Peter Pan*? If so, you will recall the "Lost Boys" from Neverland. These children, forever lost and abandoned, with only Peter to rescue them. Why Peter? Peter Pan taught an important principle that the only way to enter or escape one reality and create a new one was through imagination! "THINK of a magical thought," is just one example of hidden messages of quantum science that Walt Disney brought to life in his classics I share in my book, *What Walt Knew*.

Why is this relevant? I married a lost boy and his reality changed in an instant when he applied the supernatural laws Walt Disney taught. Sadly, my husband lost his mother as a young boy and unfortunately, she did not leave any information as to the biological father—not even a name. For 48 years my husband new nothing about his heritage and never had even a hope that he would locate his father, although the void was very real.

Needless to say, this text came as a shock to both my husband and his father. However, it's the events that happened prior that explain the mechanics of manifesting a miracle that I am very familiar with. It was not just one random stroke of the keyboard that reunite a father and son, it was a quantum cascade of feelings, thoughts, and conscious choices over time that resulted in this miraculous event.

If you have ever doubted that you are here for a purpose and that every molecule in the Universe aligns in your favor when you ask in absolute faith, the stories in this book will open your mind to the unlimited possibility of quantum leaps, also known as miracles. It is my belief that miracles are the substance of unwavering faith, the material outcome of applied free will, and supernatural creativity in the quantum realm.

Think about it. How is it possible that my husband's father was never less than two hours away? Nearly a half century went by yet did not appear in our life until the exact moment the day after Christmas 2018. A miracle manifested just weeks after my husband declared after 48 years that in 2018, this clueless mystery would be solved. How is it possible with every move my husband made to a different state, it drew our family closer and closer in proximity to his father? How could his father and siblings spend every summer at a lake home 45 minutes from our own home for 15 years?

Science has a very logical explanation called quantum entanglement, the energetic bonds of protons and electrons spinning at a distance as if they were one in the same. Spinning at the right velocity, these entangled protons may pull towards each other. There is not just a physical bond, there is a spiritual bond to our children and their children's children. Why did the company my husband works for decide to make a bold move from Michigan to Florida that brought us two hours from his father's home? There is a force bigger than you and I at work on our behalf, leading and nudging us towards our desires. That force cannot be seen but you feel it, and when you wake up to it, you learn to lean on it.

Is it ironic that my husband's father also grew up without

knowing his biological father as well? Two souls with one purpose or as many of us are programmed to believe, just the way fate would have it? Could this one-in-a-million chance really be a mere coincidence, predestiny, or was this outcome a quantum leap? Perhaps it was my husband's faith, or his dying mothers' prayer to a higher power that would guide them together at the right future time. Or, maybe it was the possibility that only the new science of quantum physics can best explain: the anatomy of miracles.

It's my belief and experience that I based my book, What Walt Knew on, which is: "to manifest a miracle the imagination must conceive an idea that requires three things working together with something much bigger than you and I could ever comprehend Faith, Trust and a little Pixie Dust (quantum particles)."

First, every miracle begins in your imagination. Walt Disney lived his life as an example of this and wanted you to understand. Has it ever crossed your mind that the Disney classics your parents read to you as a child that were supposed to put you to sleep, are actually meant to wake you up?

Individually, faith, trust, and pixie dust all have an equally important role in creating miracles in our lives. However, it is imagination that creates the catalyst for quantum leaps! I say create, because so often we refer to a miracle as something that happens randomly outside of one's self. As a follower of Christ, this was really difficult for me to grasp until I looked at the world with a quantum view. I finally understood the truth in the statement, "The Kingdom is within." Nothing happens on the outside that does not first begin in the kingdom within—the mind. Walt Disney also knew the power of this magic kingdom within that he referred to as imagination! New science called this same creative space the quantum field. This is the unseen realm where all things are possible to those that believe.

Faith—in Peter Pan's classic quote, Walt showed us the importance of having faith as the first step to access the power to create. Ancient manuscripts refer to faith as the end result of using your imagination to create something from nothing. When your creative consciousness is in alignment with a higher truth, your heart's desires manifest in the physical according to your faith. A focused, unwavering mind is the portal to manifest supernatural miracles into the natural world.

Trust—is the ability to surrender what you think you need to control and accept with ease that the possibility is already an actuality. Trust is resting in the space of unknowns, being unattached to the outcome yet expecting something incredible. This is also the quantum law of nonresistance, letting go and allowing God. Material cannot change material; only the supernatural can create something new from nothing. Trusting in something you can't see is risky, but it is also a choice.

Pixie Dust is light energy—photons! These are the infinitely endless particles of creative energy we find in quantum space that form and hold everything together. This subatomic power is what forms what you can see and touch from your creative consciousness. This light energy is at work in us and through us and begins at the moment of conception. What Walt Disney knew is that the light that has always been with you is critical to manifesting miracles on earth. Quantum particles are the building blocks of everything you see, feel, and touch. These three things—faith, trust, and pixie dust—are the foundation to understanding how to manifest a miracle. But first, you must wake up to the power of your imagination.

My husband's journey to find his father is just one of many miracles I have witnessed applying the above three things over and over in many lives, including my own! I have seen firsthand bank accounts double within less than 30 days, cancer cells disappear, cardiologists speechless, being at the right place and the right time, and the wrong place at the right time. The right people appear at just the right time to provide everything from a word to a connection or an idea. Visions and dreams are the norm when you operate out of imagination. Every single time I have applied these three things, my faith, my trust and a little pixie dust, I create the outcome I desired. You can, too!

If it's that easy, why doesn't everyone get a miracle? Why did it take 48 years for my husband to find his father? I'm sure he questioned God and his faith, wondering why his mother had to die at such a young age, leaving three young boys alone to fend for themselves. Where was the miracle when all he ever wanted was to know who the hell he was and where he came from, always questioning, "Am I enough?"

Maybe you have lost trust after asking, "Why did the business fail, the husband or wife cheat, the diagnosis from your doctor, the child born disabled." I have asked myself some of these exact questions until the day I woke up. I awakened to the truth that the life I create is a choice. Sometimes life makes sense, but the majority doesn't until you are able to connect the dots. Your words, environment, friends, beliefs, and actions are sending signals to the quantum field of imagination and sending you back exactly what you ask. Ask and you shall receive. The imagination doesn't choose, you do.

Have you ever reflected on a situation that needed a miracle and thought, if I only knew what I know now? You did! You simply were not awake to see it. The Wright Brothers did not change the laws of physics, they saw an opportunity that had always had the possibility, it just had to manifest out of an imagination! That's science, the real miracle, to take an impossible idea and create something totally new. Walt Disney loved to do the impossible.

I have proven in my own life; this technology can be applied to any situation or request that seems impossible. Any situation or idea with the combination of science and spirituality can manifest miracles. So much so that I have become obsessed with sharing this information with the masses, because it's not just for me. The keys to manifest miracles are grounded in supernatural laws that govern our world that every human has access to. There is "nothing new under the sun." The same atmosphere and gravity that carries an aircraft into the air is the same as it was 10,000 years ago. The only thing that changed was our thinking. What we thought was the miracle of flight not that long ago had all the elements already in existence. Nothing new was created, it simply manifested into this reality through a human imagination. So the question is not "is it possible?" The challenge is waking up to the reality that many of the things you thought you knew as true are no longer reliable. Even more advancements are already possibilities in the quantum field, waiting for us to access them.

A great example of this is healthcare. As a licensed Natural Doctor, I witness the power of a patient's thoughts, feelings, and beliefs daily. What you expect, you get. When you think of a miracle, do you often assume a life or death situation overcome by unbelievable odds? Things like spontaneous remissions, near death experiences, would-be fatal accidents and the list goes on…or, are you assuming the worst case scenario? If a miracle is not a random act of kindness from the "gods," what determines who manifests one or not?

Let's look at it from a purely scientific view.

The truth is every cell in our body has the ability to heal itself, every organ, even the organs we were told could not (so brain tissue, spinal cord tissue, heart tissue, pancreatic tissue)—all now are documented with the ability to heal themselves if they are given the right environment. The environment needed to manifest a miracle is directly connected to thoughts, feelings and emotions, and how we feel about this world. This includes the meanings we attach to these feelings, which arise from a database of programmed memories and belief systems. Remember everything, not just things but also circumstances are photons; the building blocks of your reality that vibrate at certain frequencies. These frequencies are the signals to the quantum field that direct your possibility into reality. Think about it like a movie on TV. If you don't like the movie, you don't throw out the TV, you change the channel. If you are diagnosed with a life-threatening disease, focus on the outcome you want to create instead of the fear that naturally will arise.

We live in fear because we were programmed to fear. Fear is a form of stress, and the stress of fear is what steals the life from our bodies, because it is a very low-frequency feeling. Your body is already a walking miracle and able to heal and reproduce new healthy cells all the time. This is where trust, faith and pixie dust play a major role of quantum healing. You must trust your body, have faith in the power of your thoughts and feelings, and allow the pixie dust swirling in the quantum field to collapse into the reality you imagine. Turn the channel on low-frequency thoughts and feelings to those of love and gratitude. These higher frequencies have the supernatural ability to enter the quantum field and reprogram reality.

Would you agree that creating something from nothing is a miracle? You do this every single day. Miracles are always within reach. However, they cannot be reached with a material mind. Your heart beats without your control. Your lungs take in oxygen without your control. Your cells are dying and reproducing new healthy ones right now. The ONLY thing you can control is the mind. The fact that your mind is directly linked to the quantum field and that you have the power within to create your own reality, and this is the greatest miracle of all.

About the Author

Dr. Carla Burns, PhD

Carla is a faith based, Master level mentor and inspirational speaker with her podcast "Claim Your Power," recently completing her PhD in Quantum Integrative Medicine, and the publishing of her book, *What Walt Knew*. Carla Burns has helped thousands worldwide achieve personal success. Carla coaches within the network marketing industry as both a top seven-figure earner as well as wellness product development expert. She has also been featured multiple times in *Success from Home Magazine*.

Over the past 10 years, Carla has built a team of over 100,000 independent distributors and millions of happy customers throughout the globe. She currently leads this team expanding over 21 countries with total sales in the billions.

Dr. Carla is an imagination master and voice of new creative thinking.

Contact Information:

Website: DrCarlaBurns.com
QiVibe App CEO/developer
Email: DrCarlaBurns@gmail.com
Instagram: DrCarlaBurns
Facebook: @officialCarlaBurns

POPEYE'S SPINACH AND THE ECDYSTEROIDS/BENZOXAZINOIDS— THE TEAM THAT GENERATES MIRACLES CALLED "HAPPY AND HEALTHY"

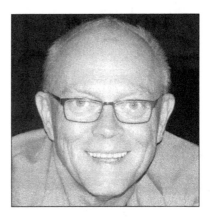

Dr. Stefan Rau

What's so great about miracles?

Miracles don't seem to happen every day. Often, they are something we cannot explain with the old scientific methods. And if we could study them and discover their secret, they would not be miracles after all. Fortunately modern science is unveiling more and more the fact that we actually can replicate and create miracles and that the old science had us blind-folded to keep us dependent and in fear.

There are a number of phenomena that would be called miracles, such as essential aromatic oils (we are still unable to explain their ways to function in all details), full spectrum CBD oil, whole-spectrum, Seed of Hope oil, and the entourage effect (the interaction of cannabinoids and terpenes are miraculous) or the brain-gut-microbiome-axis (we will probably never be able to decipher the microbiome and its significance for health and especially for our brain).

Have you ever heard of Ecdysteroids (Ecdysterone) or Benzoxazinoids (6-MBOA)? No? Both substances are found in plants and animals, and they are miracle workers, because of the astounding positive effect on the human health. Both influence neurotransmitters that are dependent on them, such as the happy hormones such as serotonin, melatonin, and others.

Let's start at the very core of this miracle.

Popeye, Spinach, and the Ecdysteroids

A friend of mine asked me last year: "Have you ever heard of ecdysterone and do you know that it has something to do with serotonin?" I looked at him a little surprised and said, "Are you kidding me?!?"

Well, I should probably mention here that I graduated with a diploma thesis in human biology about ecdysteroids at the Institute of Human Biology in Marburg, Germany in 1986. Title of my thesis was "Investigations and content of ecdysteroids in the parasite porcine roundworm *Ascaris suum*." The essential role of ecdysteroids in combating filarial parasites was already discussed, researched, and known at that time!

Ecdysteroids are insect molting hormones and essential for metamorphosis, the incredible transformation from a larva (the fly version of a caterpillar), to a pupa (the fly version of a cocoon) and finally, to an adult fly. During my studies I was already wondering why a caterpillar and a butterfly, although they have completely identical DNA, look so different. Environmental influences such as nutrition are the reason and key to evolve healthy from the egg into adult life.

Serotonin, sometimes called the 'happiness hormone' in humans, has an essential role in both humans and insects, regulating memory, appetite, sleep, and behavior. When we disrupted the function of the serotonin-producing neurons in flies, the level of ecdysteroid was reduced and that resulted in delayed development. Researchers hypothesized that with a normal diet, serotonin is released by these neurons into the ecdysteroid-producing organ of flies. So, we found that in fruit flies the happiness hormone serotonin helps to regulate the timing of developmental states in a nutrient-dependent manner.

The Medical Clinic of the University of Marburg, Germany was the first university at the time to establish the Department of Human Biology. Lab research was led and conducted by Prof. Peter Karlson under the supervision of Prof. Jan Koolman. Prof. Peter Karlson was a student of Prof. Butenandt, who received the Nobel Prize in Chemistry in 1939 for the identification of the sex hormones estrogen, progesterone, and androsterone. Together, they researched ecdysteroids, and Prof. Peter Karlson was the first who isolated and crystallized ecdysteroids in the laboratory in 1959. It was Prof. Karlson who first created the term "pheromones," which we all know that they influence how we behave and feel for each other—whether it is, for example, sexual arousal or aggression.

Now, what has all this to do with Popeye?

The character of Popeye first appeared in the strip Thimble Theatre 90 years ago on January 17, 1929. Since I am now well into middle age, I myself grew up with Popeye cartoons, and I enjoyed them dearly. Popeye's word are still sounding in my head:

"I'm strong to the finish, cause I eats me spinach..."

Without knowing where the information came from, we all believed for decades that spinach was pushed as the superfood of its time (in the1930s), and apparently Popeye helped to increase American consumption of spinach by an entire 30%. Popeye was a role model and center of the marketing campaign. Children still hear parents say, "Eat your spinach"—for its iron content—"so you can grow tall and strong." A lot of people also believed that spinach was mistakenly chosen as the super-strength giving food, as its iron content had been overrated in the early nineteenth century by some scientists, that were researching spinach. They misplaced the decimal while doing their calculations, thus giving spinach an iron content apparently ten times its actual amount!

According to the work of Mike Sutton in 2010 published in the Internet Journal of Criminology, the original error was not due to a misplaced decimal point, but more likely the result of bad scientific practice. Furthermore, Sutton claims that Popeye wasn't eating the spinach for its iron content anyway, but for its rich Vitamin A content—that's at least the case according to Popeye's creator, E.C. Segar. Although vitamin A is very important for development and growth, and it would help Popeye to stay strong, it could not be the reason for such muscle boost.

In 2011, scientists discovered that nitrates are the true energy-boosting ingredient in vegetables, and they suspected that eating a bowl of spinach (706-2013 mg Nitrate/kg spinach) per day makes your muscles "profoundly" more efficient. In fact, nitrates, abundant in leafy green vegetables, boost the mitochondria, the powerhouses in our cells, which produce the needed energy. "It is a fuel additive for your muscles—nitrate makes muscles run much more smoothly and efficiently. Nitrates have a profound and significant effect." This just shows that Popeye's projection has been all along correct," said the lead author Dr. Weitzberg of the Karolinska Institut in Sweden. According to his study, nitric oxide is an important molecule, which opens up blood vessels, lowers blood pressure, and improves circulation.

The obtained research results indicate that other green vegetables like arugula (4354 mg Nitrate/kg), celery (1496 mg Nitrate/kg), or lettuce (1264 mg Nitrate/kg) also contain significant amounts of nitrate in their composition. Which means that spinach (706-2013 mg Nitrate/kg) represents a relatively significant and acceptable amount of needed nitrates for the human body.

The main question remains: "Why did Popeye eat spinach to be that strong and not just arugula or celery?"

There is no doubt that spinach is one of the most important antioxidant-rich and nutrient dense foods on the planet. A variety of vitamins, plus Tryptophan, folic acid, and flavonoids are all present in spinach. The high consumption of spinach in Alzheimer's disease patients, which currently effects more than five million Americans (with an estimated increase to 7.7 million by 2030), are described. Spinach increased serotonin level and decreased both norepinephrine and dopamine levels in the cerebral cortex. Spinach is a brain-super-food that boosts our microbiome and has stress-reducing and anti-depressant properties due to lowering corticosterone.

Spinach and Phytoecdysteroids

Ecdyson is a steroid that was originally isolated from butterfly caterpillars as a sexual hormone. Phytoecdysteroids are similar to insect molting hormones, which I researched already in the 1980s, and some plants produce ecdysone to protect themselves from the caterpillar feeding on them.

Although phytoecdysteroids have been so far found in 6% of plant species, phytoecdysteroids are not frequent in plant species that are cultivated and used for human consumption—with the important noticeable exception of SPINACH! Spinach seeds and younger leaves contain the highest concentration of phytoecdysteroids. Quinoa contains high levels of biologically active phytoecdysteroids as well, which have been implicated by the plant to defend itself from insects, which are therefore a natural healthy plant pesticide with beneficial properties to human health.

It has been found that phytoecdysteroids balance blood pressure, have estrogenic, antiestrogenic, and androgenic effects, and do not incite virilization. Simply put, ecdysterone showed a vast amount of positive effects in regard to protect our organism against various degenerative diseases and their progression. The adaptogenic activity of ecdysterone is proven to be highly effective.

Pharmacological effects of ecdysteroids in mammals and humans

	Ecdysteroids derivatives
Antibiotic activity	-Useful in treatment of herpes zoster -Antifungal and antibacterial

Bone metabolism	-Significant Improvement in osteoarthritis and osteoporosis -Significant reduction of bone atrophy
Cell proliferation and differentiation	-Wound healing and skin regenerating -Anti-ageing effects, increases skin metabolism -Inhibits psoriasis -Treatment of burns and wounds
Glucose metabolism	-Antidiabetic effects: keeps blood sugar levels stable and minimizes the need for insulin
Cardiovascular System, Kidneys, Liver	-Prevents arteriosclerosis -Prevention of myocardial ischemia and arrhythmia. -Prevention against angiocardiopathies. -Improves renal function, stimulates hepatic functions.
Immune system	-Various immunomodulatory effects -Anti-inflammatory properties similar to cortisone -Antioxidative and free radical protection
Lipid metabolism	-Hypocholesterolemic effects -Reduces Triglycerides and LDL and simultaneously increases HDL levels
Nervous system	-Exerts a neuromodulatory action on GABA receptor -Cerebral neuron protective and antiepileptic effects -Protective effects on amnesia induced by diazepam and alcohol -Induces VEGF expression and angiogenesis in areas around ischemic brain regions
Reproduction and Development	-Ecdysteroids might increase milk production in mammals -Dietary ecdysterone or 20E enhances sexual function in rats

Phytoecdysteroids and the Anabolic Effect – Latest research found: Spinach has doping effect

In 1976, Russian scientists discovered in animal studies that spinach has influence on anabolic functions. The initial studies were done in the '70s and had not been pursued to any large extent. In fact, ecdysone is able to influence the structure of fatty cells. Dietary supplements with ecdysone-containing spinach extract decrease body fat, and at the same time increase muscle mass and strength. Today, ecdysteroids are used by many people in increasing numbers as anabolic compound.

Last year, a report was published that an increase in sport performance has been demonstrated when Ecdysterone is combined with exercises. Supported by the World Anti-Doping Agency (WADA), FU Berlin has conducted a 10-week study to further the research in this specific area:

Athletes who received ecdysterone during strength training, resulted in three times greater strength than that of the placebo group. "Knowing the long standing history of ecdysterone use, one could expect a performance increase," said Prof. Maria Parr of the FU Berlin.

Prof. Parr therefore recommended to WADA to add ecdysterone to the list of prohibited substances. Background of the study indicates that ecdysterone was used for Russian athletes to achieve greater results. Ultimately, this decision will be done by WADA. No side effects were found during the research due to the fact that ecdysteroids are structurally quite different from mammalian steroids, and they are expected not to bind to vertebrate steroid receptors.

It is highly unlikely that spinach itself will be added to the doping list. Anyone hoping to increase their performance and look like Popeye, would have to consume vast amounts of spinach. During research athletes consumed up to 800 milligrams of ecdysterone per day. This amount equals the consumption of well over 6.6 kilos of spinach daily. Referring to Popeye, who was created in 1929, Prof. Parr said, "Maybe somebody knew already something, and it was overlooked until today …"

Remembering the time when I worked at the laboratory;

Popeye and Prof. Karlson (who is considered the inventor of ecdysteroids) were a lot alike in real life. Both enjoyed to smoke a pipe, and both were sailors. During our weekly team meetings, Prof. Karlson used to talk all the time about sailing, which was his greatest passion.

Benzoxazinoids – Key to Happy and Healthy – in Maize

Have you ever heard of benzoxazinoids or 6-MBOA? In January 2019, I tested a female patient suffering from mild depression, panic attacks, and anxiety with HRV (Heart Rate Variability), and recommended her a product based on maize, containing benzoxazinoids (6-MBOA). Her condition improved within 30 minutes. She appeared more relaxed, felt energized, and when she left my clinic, she took the product with her.

Ten days later my patient called me and said, "Your product has been a miracle for my entire family! I feel fantastic and I have no more panic attacks; my husband, who is now taking it too, is not so irritable anymore, and we even have a healthier sex life. My son struggled focusing in school due to ADHD, and we gave him as well some of the product and now he can focus and relax."

This is one of many frequent feedbacks that I receive from so many of my patients.

What are benzoxazinoids?

Sixty years ago, Dr. Negus studied the breeding behavior of mice in springtime and found that food had a crucial influence on the development of the reproductive organ functions. Spinach extract, fed to female mice, increased uterine weight and stimulated the number of developing follicles in the ovaries. Sprouted wheat or maize, fed to immature females, stimulated immediate onset of estrus, as well as an increase in uterine and adrenal weights. He suggested that hormone-like substances in plants may influence reproduction in natural populations of mice. Plants have evolved sophisticated defense systems to cope with the multitude of harmful environmental conditions they face, and secondary metabolite concentrations are highest only in young tissues.

Benzoxazinoids are common Tryptophan-derived secondary metabolites in monocot plants, including the major agricultural crops maize, wheat, and rye, where it functions as defense against numerous pests and pathogens, and just like ecdysteroids this is a natural plant-pesticide with huge health benefits for us humans. Benzoxazinoids have the reputation to have pharmacological and health-protecting properties as well as positive epigenetic effects.

6-MBOA Health Benefits:

o Antifungal
o Antibacterial
o Antiviral
o Analgesic
o Anti-inflammatory
o Potential anti-cancer effect (prostate cancer)
o Anticonvulsant
o Appetite suppressor
o Anxiety (efficacy might be due to the potential effects it may have on serotonin levels)
o Depression (potentially reduces depression by directly influencing the biosynthetic pathway of biogenic amines)
o Supports the endocrine system
o Supports the reproductive system
o Acts in the area of the brain, which may be referred to as the pineal-hypothalamic- pituitary-axis (PHPA), possibly as a melatonin agonist and at the C- and B-adrenergic receptors in its own right
o Stimulates melatonin biosynthesis
o Induces TH (thyroid) activity simultaneously with a rising brain serotonin levels.

Tryptophan – The Next Superstar

Tryptophan is an essential amino acid and it is key for the production of serotonin in the body and responsible for nitrogen balance. It is also key to brain function, creates niacin, and has a role in healthy sleep. Healthy foods like spinach, eggs, seeds, nuts, etc. are natural sources for tryptophan. And tryptophan is needed to produce serotonin inside our body. Serotonin is a key essential neurotransmitter. The pharmaceutical equivalent to our healthy bodies own serotonin is called LSD, a psychedelic unpredictable and addicting drug. Ninety-five percent of serotonin is produced in our gut when our gut microbiome is functional. Tryptophan is essential to serotonin production, which in turn is the key to our own bodies melatonin production!

Serotonin is transported from the gut to the brain where the pineal gland converts serotonin (methyltryptamin) via methylation into melatonin. I am sure everyone has heard about the importance of Melatonin and that only the body-own produced Melatonin has a healthy effect and efficacy without side effects! Melatonin (N-acetyl-5-methoxy-tryptamine) is a universal molecule that is present, in humans, animals and plants. Our bodies own melatonin is 500 times stronger than DMHA (energy and stimulation), the strongest anti-oxidant AND responsible for deep *delta* sleep, which is the brainwave that is needed to build human growth hormone (HGH) and to renew, rejuvenate, and recover our physical body and our souls! Melatonin is a multifunctional factor in stress resistance, as well as in growth and development processes. Melatonin is a regulative hormone that plays as well a key-roll within reproductive processes.

Dreaming—Consciousness—Happiness—Well-Being—Health—Sleep—Strength—Mood—basically every function and functionality in our body depends on one thing: The brain-gut-microbiome-axis. The right nutrition is crucial for our health and happiness!

Personally I am very excited to now pursue research in cooperation with Eike Jordan, who supported this chapter. We will research the combination of ecdysteroids, tryptophan, and benzoxazinoids with the "Seed of Hope," as this is the potential essence to support health, and restore physical balance, resilience, and homeostasis.

About the Author

Dr. Stefan Rau, PhD

Stefan lives in Marburg, Germany. He studied biology and graduated with a university diploma in Human Biology at the Institut of Physiology of the Department of Medicine at the Philipps-University, Marburg. In the following, he studied at the Institute for Medical Microbiology and Virology Department of Molecular Oncology and the Institut of Biochemistry at the University of Giessen, where he received his PhD degree.

In the 1990s, Dr. Rau was employed for several years in the pharmaceutical and dental industry, studied economics with a focus on marketing lead to a diploma in economics with a focus on marketing in Frankfurt, Germany and teaches medical assistants in anatomy and physiology. In 1998, he founded his own company in the pain management sector, which he owned for 10 years. During this time he trained several thousand people in muscle coordination as working as an instructor for MBT Academy.

Because of his work in the pharmaceutal industy in the 2000s, he built up the Vitalforum, focused in new alternative approaches in medicine like orthomolecular medicine (how to live and to protect ourselves without drugs), building biology (effects of electrosmog on the regulation of the body), aromatherapy (the ethereal psychological and mental effects of essential oils), effectiveness of vibroacoustic sound therapy in medicine, and neurofeedback. He also worked as a product manager in the pain management and muscle stimulation sector and developed medical devices for muscle stimulation. Stefan is educated in nutritional counseling and is a certified health consultant and massage practitioner in his own clinic, where he teaches clients to regulate their body naturally.

In addition, Dr. Rau is on the medical advisory board and expert coach for heart rate variability (HRV) for the company NILAS-MV. He works in the occupational health management and carries out stress analyses with the HRV system in companies where he measured employees, analysed the effects of power napping on the autonomic nervous system and lectured about resilience.

He is a certified dyslexia and dyscalculia trainer of the Dyslexia Center Europe and has been working for several years with children and teenagers suffering from Dyslexia, ADHD and autism.

Stefan is always interested in scientific research beyond western medicine and is an international speaker lecturing on the following topics: Information and energy medicine, aromatherapy, homeostasis, stress management and resilience, heart rate variability, brain and neurotransmitters, epigenetic, brain-gut-microbiome-axis, cannabis (cannabinoids and neurotransmitters), ADHD and autism and how to get in good mood and balance with the right food.

Contact Information:

Dr. Stefan Rau
Vitalforum
Am Schuetzenplatz 2 b
Marburg, 35039
Germany
Phone +49. 17697647473
Email: vitalforum@yahoo.com

FOUNDATIONS FOR MIRACLES - THE "SEED OF HOPE"

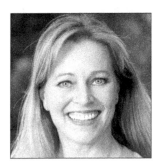 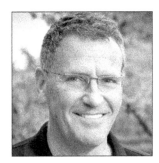

Eike Jordan & Detlef (Joe) Friede

The former member of the Board of directors of the BC College of Physicians and Surgeons, Ms. Michelle Corfield, is a core member of our team at Seed of Hope. She is a phenomenal woman, actively involved in politics, wishing to change the world back to health and balance. It is a miracle to witness more and more professionals opening up their minds and hearts in support, understanding that everyone deserves to know, understand, and have HEALTH(Y) CHOICES.

Michelle has had her share of hardship and adversity as a First Nations woman, a woman in business and politics, and as a single mother. Her son, Kyle almost died and had a long journey back to health from an autoimmune disease, and her daughter Claire suffered from epilepsy. In the face of her children's illnesses, Michelle has dedicated her life to reinstate balance and common sense.

Only through the wonderful application of indigenous and native herbs, and the wisdom of ancient healing, the recovery of Kyle started to take place. The invasive last three centuries had left scars in the First Nations perception of self, took away healthy and balanced nutrition, traditional education and ancient knowledge. And similar events happened all around the world in other nations too—the manipulation away from knowing, healing and family and shifting to fear, dependency, control, and sickness.

3-D-Healing was the first tool to initiate the healing process by non-invasively removing the negative emotions, feelings, thoughts, and beliefs. Healing past life hangovers, and within ceremony to reconnect with the spiritual realm. From here happiness and hope came back. Now we added the nutritional education to replenish the body.

Fortunately, Michelle's sister had kept the family secrets about indigenous herbs, which we now combine with the Seed of Hope and we call it Vital4Health.

So, what exactly is the Seed of Hope? And why do we need it as foundation for miracles?

In 3-D-Healing we learn that our existence is a synergistic function between the physical, emotional, and energetic body. Within our physical body we have a variety of systems like the respiratory system, the cardiovascular system, the lymphatic system, and many more including the endocannabinoid system (ECS).

There is a lot of confusion around cannabis due to the legal manipulations of the past century. I would like to take away all your fears and share some essential scientific knowledge here, mainly composed by Dr. Stefan Rau, PhD:

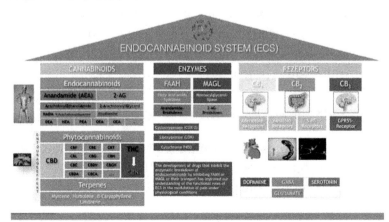

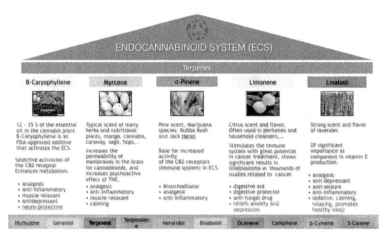

Our body builds the endocannabinoid system already at Day 16 of gestation! It is the most important regulatory system within the living body to support the immune system, the brain, the nervous system, the digestive system—it is essential all throughout! Everybody has the ECS, which continuously regulates important physiological functions like appetite, emotional responses, metabolism, mood, sleep patterns, memory, immune response, social interaction, and so much more. When a mother breastfeeds her child, she produces endocannabinoids and these are key to the child's development, as research has shown.

The ECS a key factor to reduce stress: endocannabinoid signaling reduces the activity of hypothalamic-pituitary-adrenal pathways (HPA-axis) via actions in specific brain regions by influencing the activation of neurotransmitters—such as serotonin, GABA, glutamate and dopamine. One of the main functions of the ECS is to modulate mitochondrial function and its neuro-protective properties.

The three functional components of the ECS are:

o   Cannabinoids / Endocannabinoids (Anandamide, 2-AG)
o   Cannabinoid Receptors (CB1, CB2, CB3)
o   Enzymes that break down / create cannabinoids

The three above components work together to regulate the body's functions and enable the needed adjustments when an imbalance occurs. Since the ECS functions as a retrograde system, it has direct influence on the neurotransmitters. Errors in the ECS can result in neurological disorders or can influence mental illness as a result of miscommunication within the neurotransmitters. Therefore, the conclusion is that by treating / nourishing the ECS directly the curative effect is greater than addressing individual neurotransmitters only.

The ECS also regulates intestinal functions. The brain-gut-microbiome axis is our "second brain." A multitude of studies has shown the connection between the ECS and the microbiome. When we modulate the gut microbiota for example by using probiotics, we find that the ECS gets altered, too. A new study of the American Society for Microbiology investigates the relationship between microbiota and the ECS:

The ECS appears to be the universal master regulatory system in our body!

Phyto-Cannabinoids and Terpenes (see graphics 1 & 2)

Cannabis Sativa (hemp) differs from medicinal C. sativa, since it contains only few levels of Δ9-THC and high levels of CBD and related non-psychoactive compounds. Cannabis Sativa has a long history as a medicinal plant and was fundamental in the discovery of the endocannabinoid system (ECS).

From prehistoric sites in ancient China and Nordic Viking historic ships show that cannabis has been used across the world for ages. Cannabis and its use originated thousands of years ago in Asia and has since found its way to many regions of the world, eventually spreading to the North and South Americas. It was widely used for medicinal and spiritual purposes. For example, Vikings and medieval Germans used cannabis for relieving pain after battle, during childbirth, and for toothaches.

"The idea that this is an evil drug is a very recent construction," and the fact that it is illegal is a "historical anomaly," Warf, professor at the University of Kansas, said. Marijuana has been legal in many regions of the world for most of its history.

Its high nutritional and pharmacological values, its applications and potentialities are not only circumscribed to the biological activities of the full spectrum synergies of cannabinoids. There are over 600 different compounds found in the Cannabis Sativa L plant. More than 100 of them are so called phyto-cannabinoids, which are potential candidates for neurodegenerative disease treatment.

A plethora of other bioactive molecules exists within the cannabis plant beyond just cannabinoids. They are so called terpenes: flavonoids and terpenoids. These compounds are not only responsible for the flavor and smell of the strain. They work synergistically within the full spectrum of cannabinoids in what is known as the "entourage effect."

Terpenes have some remarkable effects on humans, and the symbiotic relationship between humanity and plants is a miracle. Each terpene by itself affects humans in specific ways, even though we don't exactly understand this mechanism. Terpenes target various receptors and neurotransmitters, with the most well known being β-caryophyllene, α-Pinene, β-Myrcene, Linalool and Limonene. Terpenes engage our system to respond actively and assist in bringing to the body to the healthy state of homeostasis. Many medical experts believe that terpenes can help ward off mental disorders like anxieties and depression. However, different terpenes have varying effects, and each effect of the terpenes is a miracle by itself!

The cannabis plant family is super potent due to the fact that the ingredients interact synergistically with each other to balance the body to perfection.

The THC-CBD-CBN-Connection

The cannabis plant and its constituents have been the focus of extensive chemical and biological research for almost half a century since the discovery of the chemical structures of its two major active constituents: the psychoactive THC and the non-psychoactive CBD. The cannabis plant itself neither produces THC or CBD, but its precursors called phenolic acids. These phenolic acids are unstable chemical connections that slowly convert from CBDA to CBD and from THCA to THC.

Although quite a lot is already known about the medicinal as well as adverse effects of THC and the positive medicinal effects of CBD on several disorders, neither pathways of the phyto-cannabinoid biosynthesis are completely known. CBN is found in very small amounts in very young cannabis plants. CBN is a non-psychoactive conversion cannabinoid from THCA/THC. All three cannabinoids—THC, CBD, CBN—have been studied for several decades for their effects on the human health. CBD is at this point the most renown, but that is changing now as CBN appears to become the spotlight in research.

Other cannabinoids like CBG (Cannabigerol) and CBC (Cannabichromene) also show promising results in research although their medical applications have not entirely been concluded.

Cannabinol – CBN

CBN was actually the first cannabinoid to be identified by scientists at the end of the nineteenth century. Its structure was elucidated in the early 1930s by R.S. Cahn, and its chemical synthesis first achieved in 1940 in the laboratories of R. Adams in the USA and Lord Todd in the UK. CBN has a lot of medicinal properties and significant health benefits such as:

o strongly balancing and calming to the mind
o treatment of insomnia and sleep disorders
o pain relief
o anticonvulsant
o antiemetic
o antibacterial
o anti-inflammatory
o strong antioxidant
o promotes healthy growth of bones
o cancer growth inhibitor
o appetite stimulant

CBN for Sleep Disorders

According to the National Academies of Sciences, Engineering and Medicine an estimated 50 million to 70 million people in the US alone suffer from disorder of sleep and then of wakefulness as result. The prescription of sleeping drugs often leads to severe side effects. Out of 80 cannabinoids, CBN is the most powerful sedative, making it a promising treatment option for people that are suffering from sleep disorders, for example from sleep apnea and insomnia. According to Steep Hill Labs, 5mg of CBN is as effective as 10mg of diazepam, a prominent pharmaceutical sedative drug.

CBN for Pain Relief

In addition to its effectiveness as sleep aid, CBN has recently been identified as a potential painkiller. Rather than relieving pain through CB1 or CB2 receptors, CBN and THC release peptides from the capsaicin-sensory nerves and activates an alternative nerve mechanism to achieve the same ends (Zygmunt et al., 2002).

In another study by Wong and Cairns from 2019, the combination of CBD-CBN induced a longer-lasting reduction of mechanical sensitization than either compound individually by itself. CBD, CBN and their combinations act as peripheral analgesics for myofascial pain, tested in rats. These results suggest that peripheral / topical application of these non-psychoactive cannabinoids may provide analgesic relief for chronic muscle pain disorders such as fibromyalgia, TMJ disorders, etc. without any side effects.

Booker et al, 2009, conducted another study about visceral pain involving the antinociceptive effects of CBN to modify the pharmacological effect of THC, antagonizing the actions of THC. These results suggest that various constituents of this plant interact in a complex manner to modulate pain.

CBN as an Antibacterial Agent

A surprising discovery by researchers was that CBN could function as an antibiotic. In studies CBN effectively protects the cells against MRSA or methicillin-resistant-Staphylococcus-Aureus (Appendino G. et al., 2008).

CBN as Antioxidant

The ability of cannabinoids to be oxidized readily suggests that they may possess antioxidant properties and could be used as neuroprotective agents in therapeutic application. Researchers found that CBN exhibits antioxidant properties. Its oxidation profile, they found, is similar to CBD and THC, and these are very well known for being highly potent antioxidants (Karler R. et al., 1973).

CBN for Bone Healing and Healthy Growth

The ECS has been shown to have a positive influence on bone metabolism. Several phyto-cannabinoids including CBN and CBD have been reported to stimulate bone nodule formation, collagen production, and alkaline phosphatase activity in cultures of bone marrow stromal cells (Scutt, A. & Willliamson, E.M., 2007). There are also indications that CBN and other cannabinoids may be helpful in healing fractured bone tissues as well as reversing and preventing bone loss, making it of interest to scientists as a potential treatment for osteoporosis.

CBN and Cancer

The antineoplastic activity of cannabinoids was already shown in 1975 (Munson et al., 1975). Lewis lung carcinoma growth was retarded by the oral administration of CBN and THC. CBD did not show to have any effect on the tumour growth. In the same study CBN/THC significantly inhibited Friend leukemia virus—induced splenomegaly; this is like a miracle to me because I myself (Dr. Stefan Rau, PhD) worked on the pathogenesis of this virus as my PhD thesis in 1993 (Rau et al., 1993).

The antiproliferative activity of CBN in hormone dependent

and hormone independent breast cancer cell lines was shown in a study in 2007 (McAllister et al, 2007). However, it was not until the discovery of the endocannabinoid system in the early 1990s that research on the anti-carcinogenic properties of cannabinoids was supported.

Cannabinoids can have a regressive effect on proliferation, particularly through the induction of apoptosis, on invasion and metastasis, and on angiogenesis (reviews: Freimuth et al., 2010; Velasco et al., 2012)—these processes are of crucial and utmost importance in tumour progression.

Closing Thoughts by Dr. Rau on the Whole Spectrum CBD-CBN-Connection

As we can see, CBN shows great promise for a wide range of health benefits. And the combination of CBD and CBN is significantly more potent with greater benefits without the high or risk of THC. And I am positive and very hopeful that with all of the amazing full spectrum of terpenes, flavonoids and cannabinoids combined in one product we will see in the future outstanding research and curative results. This is truly the Seed of Hope!

To say it in philosophical words:

"The Whole is more than the sum of its parts."

Why Not CBD Isolate?

The most important downside of CBD isolate is what's known as the bell-shaped response curve. Although CBD isolate is effective against inflammation and anxiety disorders in human and animal testing, its effectiveness peaks at a medium dose but tapers off for higher doses AND lower doses. This means that CBD isolate has limited usefulness—because its effective rage of dosage is narrow and difficult to pinpoint for each individual. However, when scientists repeated the experiments with a full-spectrum, CBD-rich extract, researchers observed that the CBD full-spectrum becomes even more effective with higher dosage.

CBD - Miracles during the last years convinced me to be on the right track

For my family I found full spectrum CBD to be a miracle. Three years ago, our dog Holly had a significant growth on her right eye, and the veterinarian said due to its fast development and size he would prefer to surgically remove her eye and the area affected around it. We decided to give her a high concentration full spectrum CBD instead and the growth completely shrunk and has since gone.

My daughter had struggled with insomnia and full spectrum CBD helped her back to restful sleep. My father suffered from skin cancer and by applying topical full spectrum CBD it went away.

So many people that I met in my professional career from all around the world suffering from cancer, seizures, skin disorders, pain disorders, problems to focus, anxieties, sleep disorders and more all showed such significant improvements when taking full spectrum CBD. Now with our Seed of Hope, the safe and potent Whole-Spectrum-Oil, which combines all essential parts of CBD-CBN-terpenes and flavonoids, I expect to see not just health improvements but actual happy miracles to happen for everyone!

I am grateful to share the Seed of Hope with the whole world.

About the Authors

Eike Jordan

Born 1968 in Hameln, and raised in Germany near Hannover, I came in 2006 to Canada and fell immediately in love with Vancouver Island.

I had my entire life long a great passion for healing, which was initiated by my own health problems as a child. I suffered from such serious nephritis that I was scheduled for dialysis and only then my parents decided to try a "witch doctor," which was back then the highly reputable Dr. Med. Bruker (1909-2001). He instantly changed my nutrition and switched to alternative medicine and homeopathy and saved my life. My kidneys regained, and maintained, to date full function. Further, I suffered from severe scoliosis and through the great teamwork of massage, physio, and chiropractic professionals, my spine turned into an upright, high performance part of my body and I was able to become a competitive athlete.

Parental genetics aren't the best in our family, and I decided to break the streak of that imprint by actively changing not only my nutrition and physical activities but as well in researching, learning and applying methods of healing to my own body to proof their beneficial effects.

Health and happiness are my passions—this has been my greatest desire my entire life long.

I love studying and researching, and I find that there is simply no limit to learning. I completely understand my colleagues and patients stating that it is difficult to find the time and financial resources to be able to get a chance to look into all the various areas of our being.

After finishing high school, I decided to first study in Germany Massage, Balneo-, Electro-, and Low-Intensity Laser Therapy, Foot Reflexology, Medical Foot Care (now Podiatry). I became manager of Physiotherapy in our Rehab Hospital, and added specialties to my repertoire such as Rheumatology, Respiratory Therapy, Permanent Disabilities. Plant based therapies (Phyto Chemistry is so fascinating), homeopathy, constitutional medicine, Iridology, Biofeedback, Neurofeedback, Darkfield Microscopy, and Clinical Hypnotherapy, Hyperthermia Therapy, Oxygen and Ozone Therapy, Cryotherapy, Redcord Neurac, Nutrition Counselling, Esthetic Lasers, and Microcurrent Therapy are just some of my many studies and certificates.

The key essential is I found out that our human body has many different layers and parts. The three main components are our physical, emotional, and our energetic body. If any of the three are in imbalance it affects the other part as well.

Detlef Joe Friede and I feel very blessed as co-founders to have found an incredibly effective way and approach to healing within every dimension: we named it 3-D Healing.

Contact Information:

Naturally Healthy Clinic
210 Milton Street
Nanaimo, BC, V9R 2K6
Canada
Phone +1.250.755.4051
Website: www.naturallyhealthyclinic.ca
Email: eike.jordan@n-h-clinic.com

Detlef (Joe) Friede

Joe is a Certified Master Clinical Hypnotherapist & Forensic Hypnotist (mentored by Di Cherry), cofounder of 3-D-Healing. He is the President of the Canadian Hypnosis Association (2012-2020) and a Second Degree Blackbelt in German Ju Jitsu. He is a retired professional musician, serves on the Board of Directors at Vital 4 Health Ltd, and is the CFO of 3-D-Healing

Academy International Health Educator. He travels extensively in North America and Europe with his partner, Eike M. Jordan, helping people to unlock their full potential in healing or becoming a skilled and professional certified 3-D-Healing practitioner.

Contact Information:

Websites: www.naturallyhealthyclinic.ca
   www.gohypnosis.ca
   www.3-D-Healing.com
   www.canadianhypnosisassociation.ca.

MIRACLES—OR PERFECT SCIENCE?

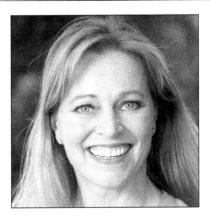

Eike Jordan

In our practice at Naturally Healthy Clinic, we are overjoyed to witness regularly miracles come true. However, we all have our own stories to tell. One thing I learned is that as the wounded healer, I can actually feel the pain my patients are experiencing.

Here is my personal miracle: As a child I faced challenges like complete kidney failure, severe scoliosis, in my early twenties I suffered nearly fatal blood poisoning, cervical cancer, two fractured C-spine vertebrae, then in my thirties, a shattered lower leg, in my forties a serious water skiing accident with severed muscles and ligaments, several concussions all throughout my life, and falling off a cliff and suffering a serious head injury in my fifties. It's a miracle I am still alive and even stronger than ever. How is that possible?

Well, let me tell you that our conventional modern medical system is a great tool, and the surgery assisted to rejoice the fractured bones in my leg. I learned though at the tender age of seven that pharmaceuticals have their limitations and do not cure, rather than causing additional problems. So, what are the alternatives? I call it 3D-Healing.

3D-Healing means the all-around approach to heal the physical, emotional, and energetic body simultaneously for curative effect. 3D-Healing entails nutrition components, restoring body functions by nourishing where deficiencies are, removing emotional trauma, enabling to learn and make informed choices, all ancient and traditional healing methods from all around the world, and hypnotherapy with the 3D-team.

Is it a miracle when I received a call on a Friday in January 2019 from one of my patients that his son in-law had been bitten by a venomous snake? He asked if I had any experience dealing with snakebites and what I might recommend as his son in-law was hospitalized in Costa Rica and struggling. After the bite occurred on Monday, the antivenom was administered but as of Friday when I received the call, his recovery had been very slow, and he was not doing well. I recommended injections with Vitamin C and oxygen, but neither were available in the third-world hospital where my patient's relative was being treated. With this situation, I tried to think outside my normal medically trained brain, to trust my intuition and go beyond my lifetime belief structure. This was completely new ground for me. I knew that my patient had experienced and witnessed incredible quantum energy based events and healings in his life. He simply believed in my abilities and because of that I decided to trust my higher Self.

I requested a picture of the man who had been bitten and received a text message with a photo of him. I focused on the picture, went out of body, and messaged my patient about what I was seeing regarding the setup of the hospital room in Costa Rica—where the bed was located in relation to the window, where the IV was located, and the location of the bite. I was seeking confirmation that I was in the correct place. My patient asked his daughter about the setup of the hospital room. Her description confirmed to me that I was in the right place and seeing the correct patient.

I had never treated snake venom before. The thought that came to my mind was to turn the tails of the molecules of the venom, stabilize the heart, bring in oxygen, and tell his soul to stay and not give up. At some point I felt a change back to health was taking place and messaged my patient that I felt that his son in-law was over the hump. I felt he was improving but was experiencing a huge headache as the toxins were processed. My patient's daughter later confirmed that her husband was having a severe headache, the first he had experienced in many years. This is called energy healing within the quantum entanglement.

Is it a miracle when we got called to the private home of Kate Lehmann? Kate is a caregiver who was unable to move for two weeks already due to most serious pain in her body. No medical explanation for her pain, and no conventional treatment helped to alleviate it and regain mobility. Somehow, she found us and called for help. One 3D-Healing treatment and she was walking again and back to work. That was in February 2019. Kate says, "This 3D-Healing is so powerful; it saved my life! I couldn't have stayed in this for any longer, it was literally killing me."

Is it a miracle when a management professional comes into our clinic in summer 2019, suffering from pain on a scale of 1 to 10 being often even a 12 and unbearable? She had gone through a hysterectomy in 2012 and ever since suffered this intense pain. She went through the entire medical system and dozens of examinations and no medical professional found the cause. All they offered at the time was that she needed to take antidepressants. She said she was not depressed, and never was. And since she works within the management of our Health Authority, she knows what she is talking about. She was in a state of desperation and very frustrated. We explained 3D-Healing to her she had one session. Immediately after the session, her pain was gone. A month later we received a beautiful testimonial from her, stating she has not had a single day of pain since that single 3D-Healing session. She is completely back to normal and a happy wife and mother to her children. Her testimonial is posted on the Naturally Healthy Clinic Nanaimo website.

And how about the cancer patient that came in in March 2019, being told he has reoccurring terminal cancer in his colon and three huge inoperable metastasized tumours in the liver?

With a regimen of mistletoe therapy, ozone and Vitamin IV therapy, 3D-Healing, nutrition change, Seed of Hope oil, and a few other homeopathic and phyto remedies … now what do you think has happened to him?

Well, he said he had nothing to lose. After the first month when he went to his awesome oncologist, he asked, "Eike says I cannot eat meat…what do you think about that?" The oncologist responded, "Well, I am not a nutritionist! So, I cannot give you any advice. But I can tell you that I myself am a vegan for a reason." I smiled big-time when my patient shared this with me.

Now, let me get one thing straight: I don't tell anyone to be a lifetime vegan. This is an extreme measure to counter the opposite extreme and bring the body back into balance. The physical state must be monitored with educational tools like dark-field microscopy, urine tests, HRV, and many other available test methodologies. Everyone in this world is an individual and needs and individualized adjustment. What is right for me must not be the same for my neighbor or you. Please always get your individual assessment done to find the perfect mixture to remove the cause for the dis-ease and imbalance.

Now, back to our cancer patient. In October 2019, six months after he started his treatments with us, his oncologist told him the cancer had disappeared – and throughout the entire time he has not missed a single day of work.

Our RN, Tina Johnston, joined our team in the summer of 2019. Tina says that since she started to work with our clinic and team, she feels for the first time in her career that she is actually healing and helping people. She is an extremely educated and sophisticated professional and teaches RNs at universities in Vancouver and Nanaimo.

My team colleague Rhonda Bonnici and her husband Brian have another very touching miracle to share:

Our story began on an overcast west coast November afternoon, with our very excited Rottie named Chevy. As we arrived at Seal Bay Park, I smiled at my partner with joy in my eyes and we got our dogs out of the truck to go for a pleasurable walk.

Seal Bay Park is a 642 hectares (1,585.6 acres) of biodiversity and treasured wildlife habitat, full of beautiful walking trails on the north end of Vancouver Island. I thought this is an incredibly safe place to take our beloved pets to for a walk. We let the dogs off leash to run and play. Chevy had been on this walk many times before and never strayed far from me, but immediately after I let him off the leash, his nose was to the ground and he went for a densely bushed area.

He was not listening to our calls and simply ran off. We thought that he would come back but he didn't return. My husband and I were getting extremely worried as we were an hour and a half into searching for him and the sun was setting. We called friends to come help. Then, finally someone found him. We felt so excited! That excitement soon faded: "Your dog has been hit head-on by a car. We pulled him out of a wet, icy, cold ditch where we found him after the impact. We are getting him already to the vet. Please meet us at the vet."

We rushed to the vet with tears in our eyes, and we asked the Divine to help guide us through this and make a miracle happen. When we got to the vet, we went straight to the table where Chevy was lying, sopping wet and lifeless. I immediately used my body as a blanket to cover Chevy as he was suffering from severe hyperthermia. I told him repeatedly that this was not his time to leave. "We will save you, Chevy," I whispered as I held him. At this point my husband and the vet had tried to get an IV in every leg but all his veins had collapsed, and he had stopped breathing. The vet looked at us with defeat in his eyes as he said, "This dog is not going to make it, and if we get him to breathe again, there is a great chance might be brain-dead." The vet was reluctant about making an incision into the throat so Chevy could breathe. My husband took action. "Turn your head," he said to me, took the scalpel from the vet and made the incision into Chevy's throat, and then inserted the tubing.

When finally the needed air entered Chevy's body, and his body started to warm up, his vitals started to improve. While I continued to hold him, he continued to become more and more stable. He did not move though and there was only little reaction in his eyes. The x-ray results came back with a small fracture in his back end and major swelling in the brain. All we could do was to make him as comfortable as possible for the night and pray for the swelling to decrease.

We returned to the vet in the morning. There was no change. The vet offered us to continue the care for Chevy as long as we wanted—but there was little hope for Chevy to recover as he didn't show any improvement. My husband stayed at the veterinary clinic. We continued to talk to Chevy and to tell him, "It's not your time. We will take care of you, just get better." We discussed what we should do next and the choice was clear. The only way to get Chevy through this drama was to bring him home. At home we have the PERL M+ technology to help stimulate healing.

The PERL M+ is a frequency instrument also known as a PEMF/Rife machine. Frequencies are utilized to trigger the body to heal itself noninvasively and naturally by running a variety of protocols such as Trauma, Brain Function, Circulation, Inflammation, Love and Healing, and more. These frequencies work behind the scenes like the songs of the world, only at cellular level.

In our minds, we envisioned and accepted only one outcome: a fully functioning Chevy living a long, happy dog-life. We had to turn Chevy carefully every hour from side to side to help circulate the blood flow in his body. We decided to lie at night with him to comfort him as the traumas were bad, praying that this supported his healing process. On day seven, we got really worried since there was still very little movement though he was starting to be more alert. We were using a catheter twice daily to relieve the bladder and fed him orally through a syringe with water and nutrients several times a day—mostly to be able to continue to give him the painkillers. Our dining room had become his ICU and would continue to be his nursing room for the next four weeks.

With PERL frequencies running daily, we decided to reduce the medication to see if we could see some improvements. Sure enough, as soon as we reduced the numbing meds, his energy started to improve, but he still could not get up on his own.

The vet advised us to include an in-home rehab specialist who brought a harness so we could try to lift Chevy up. It had been nine days without him having a bowel movement. His digestion was crucial to get going. We started taking him outside several times during the day and tried to encourage him to use his legs. I felt that Chevy needed more energy—it was the combination of everything: our prayers, our deep love, our intent, the movement, the fresh air in the garden, the PERL—it took only a couple hours to have a very large and condensed bowel movement right in the dining room. Usually, we would have screamed and be upset, but instead we did the happy dance. It's funny how life's perspectives can change so easily.

By Day 10, our dog finally had a consistent bowel movement and performed a few steps by himself each time we took him into the yard. I looked into my dog's eyes and I saw a different soul in him than he had before the accident. Not just Chevy, but our entire family spirit had changed so positively after this accident. Day by day, week after week, Chevy started to play longer, run farther, and become a new better version of himself.

Don't stop believing! Miracles are real! They are all around us and come in many forms, some are scientifically based and some just come straight from the heart and the divine up above. And since I took the 3D-Healing Certification Course it now all makes total sense to me.

-Rhonda Bonnici.

Well, Rhonda is right. Miracles are real, and miracles are science, and we all have them inside of us and around us! It just needs at times a little help by the 3D-Healing team.

About the Author

Eike Jordan

Born 1968 in Hameln, and raised in Germany near Hannover, I came in 2006 to Canada and fell immediately in love with Vancouver Island.

I had my entire life long a great passion for healing, which was initiated by my own health problems as a child. I suffered from such serious nephritis that I was scheduled for dialysis and only then my parents decided to try a "witch doctor," which was back then the highly reputable Dr. Med. Bruker (1909-

2001). He instantly changed my nutrition and switched to alternative medicine and homeopathy and saved my life. My kidneys regained, and maintained, to date full function. Further, I suffered from severe scoliosis and through the great teamwork of massage, physio, and chiropractic professionals, my spine turned into an upright, high performance part of my body and I was able to become a competitive athlete.

Parental genetics aren't the best in our family, and I decided to break the streak of that imprint by actively changing not only my nutrition and physical activities but as well in researching, learning and applying methods of healing to my own body to proof their beneficial effects.

Health and happiness are my passions—this has been my greatest desire my entire life long.

I love studying and researching, and I find that there is simply no limit to learning. I completely understand my colleagues and patients stating that it is difficult to find the time and financial resources to be able to get a chance to look into all the various areas of our being.

After finishing high school, I decided to first study in Germany Massage, Balneo-, Electro-, and Low-Intensity Laser Therapy, Foot Reflexology, Medical Foot Care (now Podiatry). I became manager of Physiotherapy in our Rehab Hospital, and added specialties to my repertoire such as Rheumatology, Respiratory Therapy, Permanent Disabilities. Plant based therapies (Phyto Chemistry is so fascinating), homeopathy, constitutional medicine, Iridology, Biofeedback, Neurofeedback, Darkfield Microscopy, and Clinical Hypnotherapy, Hyperthermia Therapy, Oxygen and Ozone Therapy, Cryotherapy, Redcord Neurac, Nutrition Counselling, Esthetic Lasers, and Microcurrent Therapy are just some of my many studies and certificates.

The key essential is I found out that our human body has many different layers and parts. The three main components are our physical, emotional, and our energetic body. If any of the three are in imbalance it affects the other part as well.

Detlef Joe Friede and I feel very blessed as co-founders to have found an incredibly effective way and approach to healing within every dimension: we named it 3-D Healing.

Contact Information:

Naturally Healthy Clinic
210 Milton Street
Nanaimo, BC, V9R 2K6
Canada
Phone +1.250.755.4051
Website: www.naturallyhealthyclinic.ca
Email: eike.jordan@n-h-clinic.com

HOW TO REPLICATE MIRACLES—
THE ANCIENT ART AND SCIENCE
OF HYPNOTHERAPY

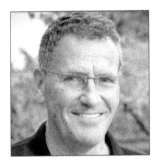 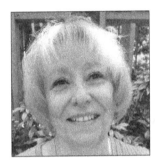

Detlef (Joe) Friede and Anita Lawrence

It is very exciting to have the opportunity to share some insights on how miracles can be created, and more importantly, they can be replicated! There are many possibilities and pathways for healing, as this wonderful book shows. Each of us studied within our given fields. We have researched ancient and modern scientific knowledge to further our ability to help our clients to heal. During our searches, we have all been intrigued by documented, so-called "miracle cures." All of us wonder, "Why did they happen? How did they happen? Why was it possible for one person to have a miraculous cure, while another succumbed to the same disease?"

Along this journey, we have encountered how to make miracles happen and even reproduce them all the time. Here is the most significant fact you need to know: each of us has the ability and choice to set the scene to create a miracle healing or change. When you work within the body's innate ability to heal itself and once a registered practitioner removes stressors and roadblocks, using the art of hypnotherapy, healing can happen. We would like to share some of our cases and results with you.

Case Study #1, facilitated by Detlef (Joe) Friede, MCH:

The following "miracle healing" occurred in 2016. My 83-year-old female client decided to not follow her physician's advice to get her right foot amputated. After a number of unsuccessful conventional treatments to enhance circulation in her leg, her physician recommended medications, which could possibly clear the artery blockage. However, when she had a CT scan on February 12, it was found that there was no blood circulation whatsoever below her right knee, resulting in gangrenous necrosis. Her physician insisted that she immediately have her leg amputated to stop the life-threatening spread of the gangrene.

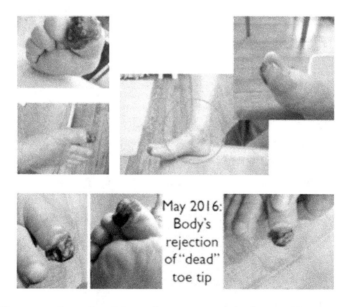

May 2016: Body's rejection of "dead" toe tip

Despite this shocking diagnosis and the medical advice, being informed and aware of the possible dangers of an advanced gangrene, my client decided to consult me instead. She stated, "Without my foot I can't drive my car, so I'd better keep my foot. Let's start to work!" She firmly planted both feet onto the "alternative pathway," fully trusting the process, and moreover having the desire to take back full control over her MIND and BODY. So, despite all medical advice, we started to work by stimulating the healing process in her body. Her physician had many concerns!

Well, her story ends with success. Here is a quick synopsis of her healing process, along with a few images. Similar to Dr. Joe Dispenza's amazing story of fully reconstructing his spine within meditation, it was vital that we prepared her body to create an internal environment conducive to healing. I stimulated her body within hypnotherapy, channeled quantum field energy, and removed unwanted blockages. Then I suggested the dead flesh on her large toe to gently release from her body. Please note that NO prescribed medication was taken from the moment on when we started working together. Only full spectrum CBD oil was administered in conjunction with hypnotherapy and energy work.

Within the light state of trance, supporting her goal to "keep that foot," the client's state of mind and dedication were reinforced utilizing hypnotic suggestions, making it easy for her to follow the detailed and specially tailored 3-D-healing protocol, including pain management. Her body responded right away and began to miraculously heal. Remember that the February 12th, 2016 CT scan revealed no blood circulation below her right knee. After my intervention photos clearly show, the new skin started to build underneath the "dead" tip of the toe, indicating there was now blood circulation to her lower leg and foot.

Surgery to take tip of the toe, May 31st, 2016

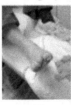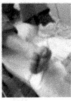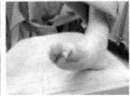

Although her family physician had not been in agreement with my client's decision, he had respected her choice. On May 31, in a deep state of trance and without any anesthetics, she underwent surgery to remove the dead flesh from the tip of her toe. By the way, during this entire process, her family physician, who had

June 3rd, full blood circulation in both feet, no swelling on any level

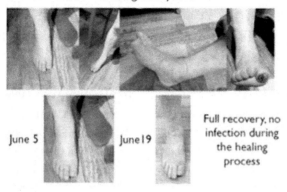

June 5

June 19

Full recovery, no infection during the healing process

initially been skeptical and rather hostile towards me, showed me increasingly more respect. By the end, though he did not understand how the healing took place, he acknowledged that it was above and beyond conventional medical explanation. As of February 2020, my client is still able to drive her car—her impetus for refusing to have her leg amputated. She is always the designated driver for her friends during all of their many excursions.

As a side note, we worked on guided imagery, projecting a new, perfectly healthy toe. This resulted in her body creating even a new toe nail where it is according to modern medicine impossible since that part had been surgically removed. This is a prime example of the power of healing utilizing the very specialized art and science of hypnotherapy and energy healing.

Case Study #2 by CHA VP Anita Lawrence, MCH:

March 4, 2006: Captain Trevor Greene of the Seaforth Highlanders was sitting on the ground with Afghan elders to discuss how Canadians could improve the quality of life by improving infrastructure. He was a peacekeeper. As a sign of respect, he had laid down his rifle and removed his helmet. Then the unthinkable happened. Without warning, and against all Afghan principles of keeping guests safe, a young village boy attacked Trevor with an ancient axe and cleaved open his skull. He was stabilized in Afghanistan, and then air-evacuated to Germany and placed in intensive care. He was in a coma, and his brain injury was so severe, they were not sure if he was going to survive.

As soon as his wife, Debbie, a friend of mine, found out about his injury, she called me and asked that I start doing distance healing on Trevor. Then she headed to Germany to be by his side. In February 2020, immediately I went into a light trance and connected with Trevor through the quantum field. What I visualized was a torn veil. That, to me meant that he could possibly die. I spoke to him and told him that Debbie was on her way, and if he could, to at least hold on until she got to him. Then I asked my spiritual helpers from the Other Side to work with me on Trevor and went into full healing mode with them.

The following day, I checked in again, and saw that the torn veil had huge basting stitches in it. He had made it through the night, though still in critical condition. But he had chosen to stay and fight. For me, it was fascinating to watch my group of spiritual miracle workers as they energetically removed debris and dead tissue from Trevor's brain, and started re-activating his neural pathways. I followed their lead. For 45 minutes each day, in trance, we worked on Trevor.

Once he was stabilized, Trevor was transported to Vancouver General Hospital. I went to the hospital a few times and performed hands-on energy healing. As everything has energy, it was important to surround Trevor with the highest vibrations possible. Debbie also brought in other holistic healers: reiki, healing touch, and quantum healers. Also, as each colour has energy, I gave her my coloured sheets to drape across him, instructing her to use her intuition as to which colour he needed each day. She filled his room with photos of their daughter Grace, his family and friends, and his travels. She brought in anything she could think of to surround him with loving, healing energy. Even Grace's baby blanket was placed over him.

Throughout this time, I continued my daily distance healing. Trevor went through some very serious moments on his road to recovery. The first cranioplasty was a failure and the skull plate was rejected. Debbie blessed and prayed over the second one, and it was not rejected. Trevor also had serious infections that caused his physicians to be extremely concerned. He was still in a coma, and I felt his waning strength and how hard was his struggle to continue to fight for his life.

I told Debbie that it would be a good thing to speak to him and tell him that if it was too difficult for him to keep fighting, then he could stop… that she and Grace would be fine. At the soul level, he needed to know they would be okay without him, and that he had her loving encouragement to cross over if he had no more strength. She said it was one of the hardest things she has ever done. But once she did this, he began to improve. He chose for the second time to keep fighting. And Debbie, despite advice from his doctors to walk away and get on with her life, chose to stay with him. His prognosis was that he would be in a permanent vegetative state and institutionalized.

Over the months that I worked with Trevor, I always said hello and goodbye, saying I would see him tomorrow. One day in my mind's eye, I saw him wave his little finger at me in goodbye. I was so excited, I called Debbie. She informed me that he had been with his physio that day and that he had moved his little finger—an OMG moment. On another occasion at around 4:00 in the afternoon, I felt him become very agitated and upset. When I checked in with Debbie, I asked her if something had happened at that time. She told me that his commanding officer had visited, and that Trevor had become quite upset, thus the "magic" of working in the quantum field. It totally reinforces that we are all connected. We just need to allow ourselves to connect on a very different level. Trevor was by this time conscious, though he had difficulty communicating and staying focused.

Trevor was moved to a facility in Langley, BC, and then on to the Centennial Centre for Mental Health and Brain Injury in Ponoka, Alberta. With Debbie at his side, he underwent numerous conventional therapies. Debbie continued to balance medical care with holistic care. Fast-forward to today. Though still unable to walk (which is his ultimate goal), Trevor is living an amazing life and inspires everyone around him. He and Debbie were married on July 24, 2010. He stood up at their wedding with the help of a brace. They also had a son.

Trevor and Debbie co-authored a book, *March Forth: The Inspiring True Story of a Canadian Soldier's Journey of Love,* Hope and Survival. He was the subject of a feature-length documentary titled *Peace Warrior,* which documented his recovery. He was also a torchbearer for the 2010 Vancouver Paralympics and is the honorary patron of the Honour House Society, a Greater Vancouver organization dedicated to helping the families of wounded Canadian soldiers. Trevor was also awarded an Honorary Doctor of Civil Laws in May 2009. All of this despite his dire prognosis that he may never come out of his coma and would probably be in a permanent vegetative state.

Hypnotherapy and the CHA

So...who says miracles of healing are a myth? Not Debbie. Not Trevor. Not me. And probably, not his doctors, physios, nurses, or numerous other holistic therapists. All I can say to Debbie and Trevor is, "Continue to march forth." All I can say to anyone else who reads their story is to never give up. Think outside of the medical box. Stop with either/or thinking and incorporate medical and holistic modalities. Above all, believe in miracles because they do happen. One of the CHA founding members, our beloved late Di Cherry, has documented case studies, where there has been bleed-throughs of past life trauma, causing severe allergic reactions in this incarnation. When the past life traumas were emotionally and energetically released, the allergies disappeared. Miraculous? Not in the world of hypnosis.

We are extremely proud that the Canadian Hypnosis Association sets the Canadian gold standard for our entire industry, thus ensuring quality care and safety for our clients. The founding members of the Society recognized that hypnotherapy is an extremely powerful healing tool. They also recognized that, undertaken by non-qualified practitioners, hypnosis had the potential to cause serious harm. The mandate of the CHA is to be the first society to set standards of practice, including rigid training curriculum, examinations, mentorship, and a clearly defined number of hours of training to attain each level of expertise. The total number of hours to be certified as a Master Clinical Hypnosis is set at 2,400 hours, which is approximately

2,395 hours more than most psychologists and psychiatrists experience during their education. In the CHA, we truly take our profession seriously.

Having set extremely high modern standards for practice, we also acknowledge that this Healing Art has been utilized since ancient times all around the world. We study the history of trance work, as well as recent scientific work published by eminent scientists such as Dr. Milton Erickson, Dr. Ernest L. Rossi, Diane Beaufort Cherrie, Gregg Braden, Dr. Joe Dispenza, Dr. Bruce Lipton and Dr. Patrick Porter, who have explored the potential healing capacity of trance work in hypnotherapy. Their wonderful research has served to enlighten the world as to the efficacy of hypnotherapy, and its role in enhancing a multitude of positive Mind – Body connections that were not previously understood in our modern society.

These scientists are the pioneers who began the process of demystifying and simplifying the science behind hypnotherapy or trance work in controlled therapeutic and clinical settings. They research and transfer the historical use of trance into our modern scientific age. As a cautionary note, we believe it is vital that everyone be made aware that there is always the possibility of instant energetic damage as a consequence of inappropriate use of words, phrases, suggestions and energy manipulation that can occur when the client is in trance. Remember, the subconscious mind is literal! Please choose your hypnotherapist very carefully and ensure valid credentials and good standing are in place.

Nowadays, hypnotherapy is employed to induce a therapeutic trance state wherein obstacles to healing are removed, and an environment is created where it is possible to create and replicate "miracles." What state of MIND has to be established within the client in order to facilitate a miracle healing? It would be easy to conclude clients should be open-minded to all possibilities. However, what about Trevor Greene, who was in a coma? In his case, Anita worked with Trevor's higher consciousness. Although he was consciously unaware, his higher consciousness was on board and working.

Some people wonder if it amplifies the effects of the work when both the client and practitioner have a shared intention of healing. Absolutely! Lynn McTaggart has written about the scientific experiments she conducted on the efficacy of intention. In her research, McTaggart has statistically and reproducibly proven the power of a group with shared intention to positively effect outcomes. It then stands to reason that, when the practitioner and their client connect an aligned intention, which gets deeply supported within hypnotherapy, the results can be miraculous.

So, why are such successes not much yet publicly known and recognized? Why are teachings and knowledge of the above-mentioned esteemed scientists, and even our CHA members, not part of any mainstream medical curricula? It is quite simple to explain: The modern medical model, historically, has given little credence to trance work. When it is taught about or mentioned within in any medical school, it has been usually allotted minimal time or importance as it is not needed for the medical board exam. It is extremely difficult to shift a pharmaceutical-based ideology to one of natural, drug-free empowerment of the client/patient. In contrast however, in China and the Middle East, pain-free major surgeries are being performed without anesthetics, simply having the patient in a deeper state of hypnosis. This is the miracle power of hypnotherapy!

It is our profound hope that with the publication of this book and with the continued scientific research and the passion for excellence by our dedicated CHA members, that so-called "Miracle Healings" will become the norm. It is time to approach healing with the recognition that there is more to us than just a body. True healing occurs when the body, mind, emotions, and soul, including the entire soul journey, are dealt with as one unit that has the *miraculous* ability to heal itself. With the intervention of a qualified 3-D healing facilitator, it can be as simple as removing the negative stressors that affect health and happiness from all sources and levels of the human being. *Then* one can truly expect miracles!

About the Authors

Detlef (Joe) Friede

Joe is a Certified Master Clinical Hypnotherapist & Forensic Hypnotist (mentored by Di Cherry), cofounder of 3-D-Healing. He is the President of the Canadian Hypnosis Association (2012-2020) and a Second Degree Blackbelt in German Ju Jitsu. He is a retired professional musician, serves on the Board of Directors at Vital 4 Health Ltd, and is the CFO of 3-D-Healing Academy International Health Educator. He travels extensively in North America and Europe with his partner, Eike M. Jordan, helping people to unlock their full potential in healing or becoming a skilled and professional certified 3-D-Healing practitioner.

Contact Information:

Websites: www.naturallyhealthyclinic.ca
www.gohypnosis.ca
www.3-D-Healing.com
www.canadianhypnosisassociation.ca.

Anita Lawrence

Anita, Vice President of CHA, is a multidimensional Certified Master Clinical Hypnotherapist, mentored by CHA founder, Di Cherry, and specialized in a variety of applications such as Past Life, Life between Lives, Soul Journey, as well as numerous energy healing modalities. She is a graduate of Arthur Findlay Spiritualist College, in Stanstead, England. Anita has served for over 20 years as Director of the Canadian Hypnotherapy Association.

Contact information:

Websites: www.anitalouiselawrence.com
www.canadianhypnosisassociation.ca.

LYME DISEASE TICKED ME OFF, BUT I BIT BACK!

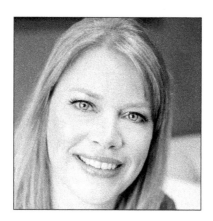

Dr. Annette Landman

Most likely my first traumatic event occurred when I was in the womb. My 16-year-old uncle died in a moped crash, and it has always been unsure if this was deliberate. In the years after that, there was a lot of loss in my family all due to traumatic accidents. My earliest recollection of the fact that my body reacts differently to injuries was when I was 12 years old. I was injured during volleyball; although nothing was broken, I did end up in a cast with torn ligaments and the healing occurred a lot slower than the specialist would have expected. When I was 18 years old, my knee started hurting without any real injury. After surgery, it was a bit of a mystery to the surgeon why I had these issues. Slowly, migraines started to occur in my life at age 19.

I am a go getter, Type A personality and just very driven to accomplish whatever comes up in my head or on my path. The decline happened over a period of years after a very traumatic divorce while living 5,000 kilometers away from my family and losing 12 people in 14 months, my health really started to take a turn for the worse. After many hospital visits, nobody could understand what was going on with me. Test after test came back with negative results. My health declined to a level where I was no longer able to get out of bed, take a shower, or use the bathroom on my own. My husband, who was self-employed and could no longer work full-time had to take care of me.

One morning, approximately nine months into not being well and getting weaker every day, my husband said to me, "I barely slept. I wasn't sure if you would still be here in the morning. We can't go on like this, something is seriously wrong." A week before this, a friend had already told me that she was getting very worried. I had lost 60 pounds, was in tremendous pain, had constant sinus infections, and had zero energy. He took me to the hospital and dropped me off. He made the decision to leave me behind so they could no longer force him to take me back home after all tests failed. He was getting desperate. Why could they not figure out what was wrong with his wife, who was always full of energy and up to something new every two weeks?

The doctor on call was very kind. He checked my information in the system and said, "We have not seen you here in 15 years, and now we see you here every two weeks. I believe you when you say that something is wrong." He did every test imaginable, even a test for Lyme disease. All tests returned negative. When he could no longer hold a bed for me, he sent me home with the message, "Please, look into Lyme disease. Our testing is very flawed, and I am suspicious that you are falling through the cracks."

Lyme disease is not really recognized in Canada and the treatment options are very limited. We found an audiobook online about Lyme disease and started listening to it. We were listening to my story, however in this case, the girl's name was Heather. After receiving a proper diagnosis of Chronic Neurological Lyme disease in San Diego, California and hearing that I was "one of the sickest people," I started Lyme disease treatments late March 2017. I chose holistic treatment, since I was not convinced that my body could handle the long-term antibiotic treatment. I was convinced that more would be gained if I would support my immune system instead of killing off Lyme bacteria. My family doctor in Canada was not willing to do anything for me, according to him Lyme disease is "the new fad disease." I needed to work on many issues: parasites, mold, heavy metals, viruses, Lyme, and other bacteria.

I started to have seizures in May. Although I did not feel them coming, I noticed that my dog Frank was alerted to their onset. He would try to nail me down on the bed or on the couch. Frank was named after a dear friend (my husband's first employer) who lost his battle with alcoholism a few months before we got the pup. One night, I had a dream that our friend Frank spoke to me and said, "It's me. I am connected to your dog. In a few minutes you are going to wake up and you have to wake up Eltjo. You will tell him to call the ambulance immediately. A massive brain seizure is coming your way." I woke up and could hear my dog, Frank, on the other side of the bedroom door, going ballistic. Never had he reacted this extreme. It was 3:00 a.m. and I did not really want to wake my husband. I was torn; who in their right mind would listen to someone in their dream? I decided to wake Eljto, told him what happened and pointed out that the dog (who we never heard during the night) was going wild.

He sat up, looked at me and asked, "How do you feel?" "I feel fine" was my answer. After a few more minutes, he decided to call the ambulance. His friend Frank had been very important to him, and he believed that this could be a message. We both felt a little weird to do so, however we live in a rural area and it would take at least 20 minutes for an ambulance to arrive. After approximately 10 minutes, I could feel some strange twitching in my face. After that, things went fast. My body went into full spasm. My whole face was cramping, and I could feel a horrible headache. The ambulance arrived and they realized that I was in bad shape. They called for backup, so they would have two people to do CPR when needed.

When they had me in the ambulance, it turned out that my local hospital was not taking any patients because they had no available beds. Something happened in my body; I could hear everything, but it was really quiet inside. Somehow, I knew that my heart was not beating. I could hear the EMT radio the local hospital and saying, "I don't care. We are coming in, and she will not make it if we have to go to the other hospital". I could hear everything, but I was not able to react. I could not move my body and felt a strange sense of peace. My life did not flash in front of me nor did I see a bright light, but I was at peace where I was. My youngest son had gone through a lot in the past year all due to my illness and since he was still living at home. My husband had so far done everything in his power to find answers, start treatments and take care of me. My father already had so much loss in his life and he recently lost his wife, his mother, and the dog.

When I imagined their hardship of dealing with my passing, I decided that I needed to try to get back. It was almost like I tried to pull myself out of some sort of strong vortex. When I opened my eyes, the EMT exclaimed, "What the fuck was all that?!" He looked bewildered. That day in the hospital it was determined that I had had a brain aneurism and my heart had stopped. Later, I learned that both were related to the Lyme bacteria in my body.

When I was sent home, my brain was very damaged. My short-term memory was very poor and my word finding skills were pretty much nonexistent. Although I am fluent in two languages, we had to pick in the morning what language we would use, since I was not able to switch between languages. On top of that, I was still struggling to put a sentence together. One day, I put the kettle on to boil some water for tea. After a while, I could hear this sound, but my brain could not connect it to anything. My husband yelled from his office, "Are you going to turn that off?" My brain could not connect that this was the sound the kettle makes when the water is boiling. At that point, my husband realized how bad things actually were.

My father flew to Canada from the Netherlands to take care of me for a month. I would get so frustrated that my language skills were so challenged. I secretly cried a lot in those months so nobody would see me. Since everyone always believed that I was some kind of strong super woman, I could not disappoint them. My Lyme disease coach stated, "We need to start to challenge your brain. If not, you might lose some functions forever. What study did you always want to follow?" For a while I had been interested in learning more about Ayurveda. I made a phone call and spoke to the dean of the local university, explaining my situation. He stated, "Do you realize that we are one of the most fast-paced educations out there? We do a lot in one year." I explained, "Perfect! That is just what I need." At least I had not lost my drive and total disregard for unrealistic expectations.

I struggled a lot in the first semester. Not realizing that with Ayurveda you learn a whole new language—Sanskrit—and the language department in my brain was already very challenged. I studied day and night and made handwritten notes from every class and then made notes of my notes—anything to help my brain to retain this. Meanwhile, I was still on my holistic program and decided to approach things with quantum biofeedback as well. When my first semester exams approached, I was an angry, frustrated, and stressed-out mess. The exams were hard, they gave me a headache, and I had no idea if I did well or not. The results came back, and I had passed and was permitted to proceed to the second semester. That summer, I was an Ayurvedic practitioner. Quantum biofeedback had been a miracle for my brain. I decided to study integrative medicine, since I needed to understand more about healing the body on the level of body, mind, and spirit.

Today, I have my own clinic. I see patients who are at the same health level as where I was a few years ago. I am so blessed that I can help them. Lyme disease was horrible, and I wish it on no one, but it was also the biggest gift to my life. Not only did it force me to slow down, I learned to explore and experience the power of meditation, healing light yoga, mindfulness, and the "three spoons per day" rule to preserve energy. My environment was a big part of getting sick. I learned that mold was a huge trigger for my body and learned how to remediate my environment. I learned how to detox my body and that you need to detox from trauma and negative thoughts as well. It is a gift that I am now able to help people who are stuck, who have tried everything, who are undiagnosed, and who are struggling. It does not matter much what your diagnosis is; there are some basic functions of the body that go out of balance and that are cause for you to become ill. That is where we start to work. I had to learn to deal with all my traumas and I decided to name it "shovel my shit." With all my clients we use quantum biofeedback to shovel the shit.

I am a new person and I don't overbook my days or weeks. I have learned to listen to my body. My drive is still there, but I only focus on things that I absolutely love. In the past few years, I have learned to eliminate people from my life who only bring drama and negativity. It is important for my health and wellness to experience life at a high frequency. Stress and negativity are low frequencies, and I don't want to have anything to do with it. Often people ask me, "How long have you had Lyme disease?" I honestly don't know, maybe almost my whole life. But when things started to fall apart on a mental and emotional level, the bacteria had a chance to take over since my immune system crashed.

After getting a second chance at living, I decided that I need to use this opportunity to help others. Nobody gets through all this to just continue living a poor lifestyle. If you don't understand that message, your health will crash again with most likely disastrous consequences. Many details of my illness are lost to me; the brain is a pretty magical organ, and I think it protected me. I had bad day after bad day with horrible migraines, neck and joint pain, TMJ, teeth that were hurting, and absolutely no energy. While talking to my husband to see how he experienced everything, I realized that I was missing a whole year. In my memories, a whole year is gone. I am so thankful to my amazing husband, Eltjo. He never gave up on me, he kept on fighting, and even though his wife had as much brain function as a vegetable, he believed that it would come back.

My recovery is a miracle; however, it did not happen spontaneously. I had to work to get better. My dog Frank is still my protector. If I overdo things, if I am stressed, or if I am sad, he shows up and steps in. My brain works a little differently. In the past I had a photographic memory, but now I really must work hard to retain information. I now know what it means to say IT'S GREAT TO BE ALIVE!"

About the Author

Dr. Annette Landman, PhD

Annette has been guided to work with clients due to her own health struggles. She has a body, mind, and spirit approach to tackle any health crisis. Her passion is to help people who have been stuck in a health crisis/chronic illness and guide them back to great health. She works with clients in person or online as a quantum health coach, biofeedback specialist, Doctor of Integrative Medicine, and Ayurvedic practitioner.

She named her clinic "My Goodness," as these words have so many positive meanings. People say it a lot because they are amazed with their progress. Annette chose this name because she wants to practice from her heart and give her "goodness," the best of herself, to her patients. She has worked with hundreds of people from all around the world. Since she narrowly survived Lyme disease, she now works with many people who have been struck by this condition and is booking great results.

Contact Information:

Email: landman.annette@gmail.com
      info@MyGoodnessClinic.com
Website: www.annettelandman.ca

THE HEALING MIRACLE OF LOVE

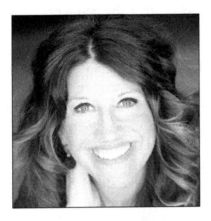

Leah Roling

My dad left and my mom raised me. She was the epitome of unconditional love, the most selfless person you would ever know. She single-handedly raised three kids on her own, never complaining. She never once said a harsh word about my father, not one. Not even for all the times I would cry and get angry with her for kicking him out. Over time I came to realize that he was an alcoholic, and completely dependent on my mom for all things. He drank his wages, and well, housework and raising kids wasn't really his thing.

How easy would it have been for my mom to be honest? It was deserved. Why couldn't they just make it work? The easy conversation would have been, "Honey, your dad was an alcoholic. He was mean, and it was unsafe for me and you kids to remain under the same roof as him." My mom didn't do easy, she did right. It was more important for her to ensure that I saw my dad through my 8-year-old eyes—pillow fights and sliding down his legs (he was 6'6" and so his legs made a pretty awesome slide). I was his little pooh. That is the memory she wanted me to keep. I now realize it was this memory that kept me focused on wanting to make him proud, which looking back translated to great achievements, successes, and an internal motivation to be better and love better every day. Who knows—had she painted this picture of an alcoholic father that wanted nothing to do with his daughter, I might not have wanted him to be part of my life.

My mom would say that she had a great life and one might even believe that it was easy since she never complained. However, nothing could be further from the truth.

At 18 months, my brother was diagnosed with spinal meningitis. The doctors told my mom that he would be in a coma for whatever remaining life he had. Luckily for my brother Bob, mom had the stubbornness of a German and the compassion and love of Mother Teresa. She told the doctors that although she appreciated their efforts, she would like to take Bob home and love him there. And love she did. It wasn't easy. He could not walk, so she hired physical therapists. He could not talk, so she hired speech pathologists. He had seizures, so she hired neurologists. The prognosis was not great but yet she loved and loved and loved. He turns 50 this July.

My sister was dropped at the age of three months. The corner of her head hit the coffee table and then she fell to the hard wood floor. She coded, received 156 stitches, and one and a half months later she could take her daughter home. I am sure that it was my mom's steadfast love that brought my sister back. She is alive and well today at 52.

My mom retired on January 18, 2018, after 50 years of service. This was also the day of her cancer diagnosis, Stage 4 lung cancer. The MRI showed a huge mass on her sacrum, with smaller masses on her liver and lungs. When the oncologist told us, I collapsed. I was every emotion in one: I was pissed, scared, and sad. I felt in that moment that I was the one dying. I looked at my mom with tears dripping from my eyes and she held me. The more I cried, the madder I got. I kept saying this just isn't fair! How can someone that gives, and gives, and has suffered so much already get this. WHY?

"How did you get here?" my mom asked. I really wasn't in the mood for rhetoric and quite frankly didn't understand the question. I said, "What do you mean?" She said, "To get to room 368 in Powell, you have to walk through Blank Children's Hospital. You want to talk about fair, go down and talk to the parents of these children and then come back and talk to me. I have experienced much. I have three beautiful children, five amazing grandchildren, wonderful friends, and memories of a lifetime. Some of those children won't see their second birthday." This is my mom. She is my miracle. This is who I had the honor, and great privilege to be raised by, loved by, and learn from.

The diagnosis was not great; her cancer was everywhere. I made it my mission to love this cancer out of her. That night my husband and I stayed up all night reading, highlighting, and putting a care plan together for her. However, even the best made plans have hurdles. Not even one week after the diagnosis, she was back in the hospital. The sacral mass shattered her hips. She lost her ability to go to the bathroom due to the nerves that were severed. We spent the next four months at John Stoddard Cancer Center. Some days she would know who I was, other days she would ask me, "Is Leah coming today?" No one thought she would ever make it out of there, let alone go home. I knew she would.

I was mad but never in front of her. I was frustrated. You hear of the stories of people that are diagnosed, plan trips, and do all the things on their bucket list. Yet, how could she? She couldn't walk. Mom was on so much pain medication; she didn't know the day of the week. Every time they had to move her, painful and worrisome tears rolled down her face. She wasn't eating, either. She was on oxygen, lying there, helpless.

I told her she would walk again and that she would go back home. But she was not convinced. It was one of the only times that I could remember she wasn't positive, and quite frankly there was no good reason to be. I told her from that moment on that it my job to worry and her job to be hopeful and believe in miracles. I wanted her to be the miracle she has always been to me.

Only one doctor would perform the surgery to cement her hip back together because of the risks. Yet, without it she would have never walked again. He said that it would be challenging.

He said that it would probably take two attempts to get it and even then, was not convinced that it would work, but he said he would try. The surgery was awful for my mom. Nothing they gave her touched the pain and yet when the doctor said he was hopeful and that it cemented nicely but she would need to have a second surgery, she said, "We can do this." She was so brave.

The second surgery was just as successful and slowly she started her healing journey. The cementing helped alleviate much of the pain and so we were able to scale back on the pain medications. This also allowed for better cognitive function and for the first time in four months she could actually think about a reality that was positive. It was miraculous.

We moved her into a short-term care facility to get her strong enough to go home. Mom amazed everyone. Her contagious joy, loving wit, and selfless kindness won the hearts of every single person she met—but I bet you knew that already.

Mom moved home a few months later and although there seemed to always be something, the good days outweighed the bad. She was able to see her grandsons play baseball, have lunches with girlfriends, get manicures, and live. Grateful and blessed have new meanings as she was able to share both Thanksgiving and Christmas with us. In June of the following year, her first grandson was getting married. Mom wanted more than anything to be able to walk Cody up the aisle at his wedding. She wanted to do it without a walker. She wanted to dance with her brothers and all of her grandchildren, and she did just that.

After the wedding, good days were fewer and replaced quickly with bad, then awful, terrifying days. She no longer responded to immunotherapy and the cancer spread to her adrenal glands and intestinal wall. The masses on her intestines caused her to bleed out, which necessitated the need for several blood transfusions weekly. The transfusions were not as easy as one might think. It required special blood to be med-flighted in since she had rare antibodies. This meant we had to get her to the hospital, which was no easy task. She had grown weak, thin, and fragile. I knew the transfusions helped; I just wasn't convinced that the pros of receiving them outweighed the cons of all the preparation.

I felt the end come closer and closer. Mom was my world; she was my everything. I was not ready even though I knew in my heart that she had suffered enough. I knew that she deserved this much-earned peace. I fought it. I loved and prayed harder. I told my energy healer that I was going to love this cancer out of her.

I felt it working. Mom hadn't had a blood transfusion for almost a month. I wanted her to see her oncologist and was positive the scan would show remission. She agreed to meet and do an MRI but did not have my same optimism. The scan results didn't, either. I asked the doctor why and how for almost two months she needed a blood transfusion twice weekly but for the last month she hadn't. She couldn't explain it and it didn't matter. I continued to love, pray, and fight—almost to my demise.

I could not sleep. I could not workout. I could not take care of my family. I was falling apart. I thought this was just the cumulation of the past years; after mom's diagnosis I went from having regular periods to menopause at 43. I needed to see Cari, my energy healer. I told her that I thought I might be anemic among many things. I could barely make it up stairs without having to sit down and find my breath. She told me she felt I was not anemic and that I was in adrenal failure, which made sense given the high level of stress that I had shouldered for 24 months. My friends and family, however, all suggested that I should be evaluated. Lab results from my doctor showed that I was incredibly anemic and that not only did I need a supplement overhaul, but a blood transfusion.

The next day, Cari came to meet my mom, it had been on the books for a couple of weeks. I decided to tell her that I got my bloodwork back and I was anemic, and that I might need a transfusion. Without missing a beat she said, "It's not yours." I didn't quite understand but knew that we would talk after her visit with my mom. As soon as Cari finished with my mom, she came to find me in the living area in the facility. I wanted to know how her visit went and what mom's state of mind was. It was certain, per usual that her state of mind was still state of care, specifically about me. Mom knew that I hadn't been doing well, and that even though I tried to keep it from her, she knew. Cari refocused me back to our initial conversation about the blood not being mine. In her way of bringing things to light, she muscle tested me. I was transfusing my blood to my mom. I immediately muscle tested YES! If there ever was an aha moment, this was it. My eyes popped open...of course, I was giving mom my blood. That's why she hadn't needed a blood transfusion, and it's why I did.

Mom always taught me that thoughts become reality. The words you say mean something. I said early on in this journey that I would love her "better," and for the time that I could, I did. Cari asked me if I wanted to continue giving away my blood and my life. I knew that my health was severely compromised, but I also understood exactly what that meant. I told Cari, "I don't think I can willingly do that knowing that with it I would compromise my mom further." She replied, "Your mom does not want you to do this for her." She then asked, "If your kids were doing this for you, would you be okay with that?" "Obviously no" was my response. I let her do her work and she created the space for me to take my blood back. She helped me find peace, acceptance, and gratitude in this miracle of miracles.

Cari visited my mom on a Tuesday. She gave me the space to take my blood back that same day. By the end of the week I started feeling better, sleeping better, and yes, I got my blood checked. My levels had returned to normal. Mom passed away the following Tuesday, one week from Cari's visit. Cari told me after mom passed that she had been ready, she just needed to make sure that I was. Even in her final week, days, and hours, she was selfless, loving and deserving of the peace she now finds in heaven.

My mom taught me a lifetime of lessons that have supported my life's work of coaching people to live their best life. I believe that everyone has the capacity to do anything they put their mind to. I believe that the answer to everything lies within us and is guided by our values and our truth. I believe in love and was taught how to love by one of the greatest. It was because I was loved that I could love my blood to her. I guess when you love someone that much, anything is possible—yes, miracles. I believe they happen in everyday love, so let's love and create miracles. Are you ready for a miracle?

About the Author

Leah Roling

I am first and foremost me! Unapologetic, imperfectly perfect me. A lucky wife and mama of three amazing boys. I am an author, speaker, entrepreneur, quantum coach, selfologist, and lover of life. I am going to let you in on a little secret: I didn't used to be me, and I didn't love my life. I used to be what everyone wanted me to be. I was a people pleaser and a worry connoisseur. I spent a good part of my life being resentful, feeling guilty, unworthy, and hating myself and my life for it. I kept thinking that if I was smarter, more athletic, more popular, and prettier, my dad would not have walked out of my life. Little did I know that this void could be filled by me and me alone.

On my journey, I have had my highs and lows. I have had awesome careers and opportunities to continue my education along the way. I picked up a Masters in Exercise Physiology, and a minor in Economics/Finance. I am certified in personal training, strength conditioning, life and quantum coaching, NLP, and Hypnosis to name a few. I am finishing up my Doctorate in Natural Medicine and have been a life learner of all things personal development. In all of it, nothing was as impactful as coaching.

When you get coaching you are challenged to get real. You are challenged to dig deep, be vulnerable, and give in. It is in this giving in, this return to self that you find yourself. You become aware of the thoughts you hold, free yourself of the secrets you keep, and learn to love and accept yourself wholeheartedly and unconditionally.

When I found coaching, I found me, and now I get to take us both into the world with a hope to inspire others to do the same. I have the privilege to empower women to rediscover their sense of self and reclaim their joy. I help my clients create an awareness around their thoughts and emotions, and shine light on the path of intention. I teach the science of neuroplasticity, quantum physics, and mindfulness to demystify the record of the past so that we can explore the map of the future.

What you want, you can have! Your thoughts become your reality and I am living proof of that. It is 100% in our control. I am blessed beyond measure to get to do the work I get to do. I am blessed to inspire and be inspired by women being curious, women searching for more, and women learning to show up authentically brilliant, self-accepting and unconditionally loving.

I am the luckiest woman in the world—and here's another little secret—so are you!

Contact Information:

Email: leah@theartofselfology.com
Telephone: (515) 865-6716
Instagram: www.instagram.com/leahroling/
Facebook: www.facebook.com/leah.roling

TURNING PAIN INTO PURPOSE: MY JOURNEY OF HEALING

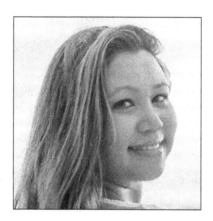

Jamie Cabaccang

My life has been through cycles of death and rebirth, death, and rebirth, death... and... rebirth.

It is through my life experiences that I have faced distressing situations. I've learned some of the hardest lessons and transformed that energy into purpose, which is evidence to the miracles that surround me in my own life.

Miracles are created through the invisible: love, pain, suffering, loss, hope and the intelligence of the universal flow of life. Sometimes it comes in the form of situations, an illness, a tragedy, or a person. These ingredients are found along the way towards becoming a miracle. In going through the process it's so hard to see the miracle being created. Think of the labor during childbirth. You're so focused on the pain that it's difficult to see anything else even when you are birthing one of life's greatest miracles—a child.

I didn't realize the people who bullied me all throughout

school and in my career were teaching me feelings of unworthiness, powerlessness, helplessness, and seeking external validation so that I could someday transform that energy into compassion. I experienced these feelings firsthand so that someday I could create a safe space for these people to heal.

Losing my unborn child brought such intense devastation with so much grief. A part of me died, too. Until recently, one of my life teachers helped my husband Rodney and I shapeshift that heavy weight of shame, loss, and responsibility we carried for so many years. It transformed into a beautiful acceptance knowing that there wasn't anything different that we could have done. Our unborn child served an intentional and everlasting purpose in the short stint of time it was in our lives. This experience birthed my relationship with my soul-husband into divine union. If it weren't for our unborn baby, all the circumstances that followed would not have happened. Life would have been very different. Now, we have the miracle of our two children, RJ and Jewel.

I didn't realize how my life would change the day my phone rang, and my son was having an allergic reaction and I could hear my son saying, "I can't breathe daddy, I can't breathe," while I could hear the fear in my husband's voice telling me it doesn't look good. It was the day I learned to appreciate the little Lego pieces my son left on the floor, the sound of his voice, his clothes laying around, and cuddling his warm, little body. He survived; thank goodness for the medics and perfect timing. It made me slow down in life, not taking my loved ones or even a simple breath for granted. And it led me to becoming a volunteer for Soulumination, a nonprofit celebrating the lives of children and parents facing life-threatening conditions by creating handmade photo gifts for families as a legacy of their loved ones.

My most recent cycle of death and rebirth has guided me towards discovering my purpose.

Being diagnosed with a painful, progressive, and disabling disease was something I definitely did NOT see any good coming out of. I started feeling really sick with various symptoms and things were just getting worse. It took months and many lab tests before my doctor diagnosed me with a chronic illness that I knew nothing about, telling me she had "lost many family members" due to my same illness.

At the time of my diagnosis, I was not in alignment with my higher self. I am a wife, mother of two, worked full-time, and was busy taking care of everyone else. I tried to carry the responsibility for everything. It was quite easy for me to put myself lower on the list of priorities. On the outside it looked like I was successful doing it all, but emotionally and spiritually I felt empty and exhausted.

I was experiencing one of the lowest points in my life.

All of this added up to me grieving my life for three months. I felt sorry for myself and stepped into the victim role. There was still so much I wanted to accomplish in this lifetime, yet I was dying on the inside as well as on the outside. This forced me to reflect on how I was spending my time and energy. Since I didn't have much energy left in me, I literally had to plan naps throughout the day and say no to things (as I was a "yes" person). I questioned everything, from how I spent my time, to whom I spent my time with, questioned my career, my environment, myself… EVERYTHING.

I went searching and searching and searching some more, but I was lost. I didn't know where to start or who to go to. I'm grateful I have a loving family who supports me, but I didn't want to worry them more or be a burden. I didn't want anyone to see me suffer. I hadn't known anyone who experienced illness like this who truly understood what I was going through. I was so lonely. How could I search for something that I didn't even know what I was looking for?

All I wanted was healing. All I wanted was answers.

The days were intensely heavy from carrying the emotions of stress, worry, anger, helplessness, and confusion. On top of that, I was in pain and getting sicker. I was lingering in the fate of the illness. It was extremely uncomfortable and not sustainable.

All the knowledge that I had at the time wasn't going to heal me.

A turning point for me was when I turned my *cant's* into *choice* and my *pain* into *purpose*. I chose to be uncomfortable experiencing new things I've never done before as long as it nourished my healing. It required me to let go and just LET BE. I opened up my mind, heart, and soul to trusting the Universe, and it was a new way of being. I traveled solo to deepen my relationship with myself. I am rarely alone and am surrounded by people all day at home and work. It was the ultimate gift of self-discovery.

Each person I connected with, I learned something new about life. Each time I connected with myself, I learned something new about me. I realized that every person I interact with is either a student or a teacher; I was either learning or sharing something. These connections introduced me to different healing modalities including sound healing, Reiki, breath work, meditation, sensory deprivation tanks, astrology, aura readings, Body Talk, crystal healing, somatic therapy, EFT, anti-inflammatory diets, natural remedies, Tibetan medicine, acupuncture, shamanic journeying, PEMF therapy, earthing and even putting a leaf under my tongue while sitting in the aura of a 1,000-year-old tree. This healing journey became a soul-fulfilling adventure!

I was fascinated and ready to integrate these learnings into my way of being. The Universe brought some of the best life teachers into my husband's and my life including Margaret Piela and Sand and Jon Symes. Through working with them, I began shifting the energy of the victim mindset. I embodied the perception of life happening *to me* to finally realizing that it was all happening *for me.* This is where I began to be the creator of my life experiences.

What I learned is that there is no one person and no one answer that could provide me with complete healing. It is a journey that you have to go on to find what works best for you, because what may work for one person—even with your same condition—may not work for everyone. This is especially true if you are searching for more natural methods to heal yourself holistically. While I appreciate modern medicine (such as the epinephrine injection that gave my son a few extra breaths before the medics arrived), I made the decision to first try healing myself naturally instead of being on steroids and chemotherapy for the rest of my life.

I finally met a doctor who gave me hope, Dr. Sharum Sharif, ND. He introduced me to the world of homeopathic remedy, which gets to the root cause of the symptoms. He told me to forget the name of the disease because it's just a label. If you heal from the root cause, you will not have any symptoms, and therefore you don't need to worry about the disease. Within less than a month, my symptoms were gone, and my energy was back.

Homeopathic remedy is energy medicine made from plants, minerals and animals diluted to its most minimal form—energy— which is invisible to the human eye. My own healing experience made me curious about how energy works, with the body's own healing powers, to bring about healing change. I saw energy practitioners, not knowing what to expect. I physically felt the energy. It's a profound experience with no words in our vocabulary to describe what I went through. There was something so healing for me as it awakened a deeper connection with myself. Just as homeopathy gets to the root cause of physical symptoms, I was tapping into the root cause of my emotional traumas and healing from within. It is the stress and emotional traumas that actually cause physical illness, and that's why holistic wellness is so crucial.

Being diagnosed with an illness led me to discover my gifts of helping others in a transformational way.

I was inspired to become a certified Reiki master to deepen my healing. I had no intention of becoming a practitioner. In giving others Reiki, I realized that I was able to help individuals in a profound way by connecting them with their truth and awakening their mind, body, and soul's intelligent ability to heal itself. I opened up my practice, Pure Reiki Wellness, and I'm typically booked out a couple months in advance.

I am a hybrid: I transform the way people live and work through designing technology and as a holistic wellness practitioner.

I am a product design leader, inventor, manager and mentor in tech. I hold many patents and product design awards.

Aside from designing technology experiences to solve problems, I also design safe spaces that honor vulnerability for employees to be heard and hear others without judgement through connecting with people individually and cultivating support groups. I facilitate feelings meetings that allow people to grow from beyond the label of co-worker to your fellow human being you can relate to and have compassion for. I hear the struggles and see the masks people put on in order to hide their authenticity and be accepted, powerful, seen, promoted, liked, or feel a sense of belonging, validation, and support.

As an energy, mind and soul practitioner, I hear the raw stories behind the mask. The root cause of the existing challenges. The "why." The needs and fears. This suffering can be disabling and detrimental to expressing one's self and living one's purpose. Most times, these needs and fears stem from our experiences as children. We stuff those emotions, so we don't have to deal with them. We avoid them and keep ourselves distracted as if they didn't exist. Why? It's easier to numb ourselves from feeling. It is easier to protect our hearts from giving and receiving love. If we build a wall to protect our hearts, then no one could hurt us.

We find ways to not fully express those emotional energies. When a situation arises, it can cause emotional triggers that are not only about the current situation, yet it is a deep felt emotion being expressed from the past. This could be a very painful cycle. What we don't realize is that when we begin to feel, then we begin to heal. With these intelligent human capabilities, you are meant to feel these emotions because it's information to help you realize when you are on your soul's true path and when you're not.

It is through my love for designing transformative experiences, my compassion for people, and my healing journey of discovering my inner essence that have led me to birth the bridge between the two communities, which I call Techies + Wellness.

Because I am embedded in both the tech and wellness worlds, I live and speak the language of both. Both communities need each other, and I bring them together naturally. I am here to create patterns that have never existed before. We empower tech professionals by helping them discover their inner essence, improving their well being from deep within through our thoughtfully curated event experiences and transformative retreats. We are especially for those who are ready to step fully into their authentic selves. Those who are healing. Those who are stuck and are open to deepening their relationship with themselves and create shifts in their lives. Those who are saying "No more. No fucking more," and are sick and tired of being sick and tired.

Our growing community includes employees from Microsoft, Apple, Google, Facebook, Amazon, Intel, Oracle, Boeing, Pinterest, startups, and many more. Everyone is welcome to join us—techie and non-techie alike. It is important to bring holistic wellness and mindfulness into the tech community because these are the people who are building our future. They are engineering the world around us, but what about engineering their world within? When they have a deeper connection with themselves, it can lead them to a life and career that is an energetic match with their passions and true calling.

The more we can improve the lives of people creating our future, the better our world will be.

In going through the process of death and rebirth, there's that peak that you reach when you feel like the worst thing in the world is happening to you. Emotions are your soul's way of communicating what's true for you. It's painful; it stings, and you may feel helpless and lonely. Feel it. Experience it. This feeling is temporary. You have choice. Observe and notice the lessons you are learning and the things for which you are grateful.

This disconnect with yourself all happens for a greater reason. It can sometimes become so agonizing that it leaves you no other choice but to reconnect inward so that you can connect with the world around you in a more meaningful way. It is through this process that miracles are created! The more you ignore your emotions, the louder and more obvious it will become. Your wellbeing, situations, and relationships in your life are a reflection of how you are honoring yourself and your needs.

As I reflect on my experiences and the people throughout my life, they are all beautifully threaded together. They each contribute to learning different perspectives about myself and teach me the lessons I am here to learn. My awakening is also teaching me to unlearn the stories that no longer serve me. These fuel the inspiration for me to create life experiences with purpose and thoughtful intention. I've had to lose myself in order to find my inner wisdom. With each cycle, I am faced with having to dig deeper into my truth. My soul's calling. My higher self. The purest essence of me. Each time I go through this cycle, I grow a closer relationship with myself and a miracle is birthed. My entire life is a miracle. Yours is too, if you choose to see it that way.

About the Author

Jamie Cabaccang

Jamie is an award-winning Product Design Leader, Founder of Techies + Wellness, and a Certified Reiki Master at Pure Reiki Wellness. She worked at Microsoft for over 10 years and currently works at Pinterest. She is compassionate about helping others improve the way they live and work through both transformative technology and holistic wellness.

Techies + Wellness is a bridge between the tech and wellness communities on a mission to empower tech professionals, improving their well being from within by bringing holistic wellness resources, event experiences, and transformative retreats. Their growing community includes tech employees from Microsoft, Apple, Google, Facebook, Amazon, Intel, Oracle, Pinterest, tech startups, and more. Techies + Wellness has been a part of hundreds of life journeys thus far, connecting individuals to their own inner wisdom, guiding them on their path to self-discovery, authentic self-expression, and honoring their true calling. Jamie believes that the more we can improve the lives of people creating our future, the better our world will be.

Contact Information:

Learn more about Jamie
www.jamiecabaccang.com

Techies + Wellness
Holistic wellness event experiences and transformative retreats
www.techiesandwellness.com
Join our community on Facebook and Instagram @techiesandwellness
hello@techiesandwellness.com

Pure Reiki Wellness
Book an individual energy, mind and soul session with Jamie
www.facebook.com/purereikiwellness
purereikiwellness@outlook.com

LIFE IS A CHOICE...
ANYTHING IS POSSIBLE IF YOU
ALLOW MIRACLES TO HAPPEN

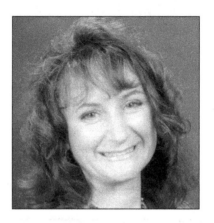

Diane McKee

In March of 2017, I faced my third instance of a near-death experience. As I lay curled in a ball, unable to move in the ICU, I felt numb to the noises and chaos surrounding me. I was a hot mess. With a chronic fever from sepsis, my joints were frozen, my strength in my muscles diminished, and I suffered extreme weakness from months of nutritional deprivation and dehydration. My lungs were partially collapsed and inflamed, making it difficult to breathe. As if that were not enough, my spleen had been enlarged for months, inflammation surrounded the pericardium of my heart, and my kidneys and liver were failing. Could this really be the end for me?

I lay dying, thinking I would never survive. That is when I heard a distant voice ask, "Do you want to stay or go?" I replied, "I feel something is not yet complete with the purpose of why I am here. I would like to stay." The voice then responded, "If you are to stay, you are to become hope and inspiration as you move forward." Wow, what a powerful message! I had been given the choice of LIFE.

Immediately after the conversation, I found myself being wheeled into surgery for a kidney biopsy. The procedure determined that my kidneys were failing due to acquiring systemic lupus, a severe autoimmune disorder. Next, heart surgery was required to release the pressure of inflammation around my heart.

Without a shadow of a doubt, I had been gifted with the miracle of life. Anything is possible! I felt giddy like a child and felt joy entering my heart knowing I was alive. At this point, I realized I had just been provided an opportunity for a new beginning. Deep within myself, I knew I had to do everything I could to regain my body's strength and vitality to fulfill my new life's purpose of bringing forth hope and inspiration.

After 10 days in the ICU, a rehabilitation center was carefully selected in the middle of a state forest. The ideal healing environment became more important than money, with sunlight streaming from a large window. My family advocated for at least 30 days of treatment to relearn how to stand, place one foot in front of the other, lift my arms, and move my fingers, toes, arms, legs and body. Most of my muscles had lost their memory of how to function. I had no idea it was possible for muscles to forget how to do that! My body did not remember how to breathe due to chronically collapsed lungs. The simple acts of sneezing, coughing, and yawning felt impossible at times. My chest and ribcage ached with each breath.

My heart space became so overwhelmed by immense gratitude and deep appreciation for what was left of my body that tears flowed from my eyes. As my attention was refocused, I recognized the importance of gratitude for what NOW worked instead of what was gone. Also, I realized the importance of forgiving myself for allowing my body to get to this point. Wow, another awareness from the unknown! I started loving my frail-looking body exactly as it was.

Feeble muscles and fat hung loosely from my bones and I was in a state of complete dependency. Each day, nursing assistants fed me an abundance of proteins and nutrients with a little salt placed into my water to enable my body to hydrate. Loving, compassionate nurses carted me around in a wheelchair to meals, therapy, and back and forth to a scale to monitor my weight. In addition, physical and occupational therapists worked with me to relearn how to breathe, move, and begin to care for myself again.

The high dosages of steroid and chemo-type medications created severe side effects. I could not sleep, regulate the heat of my body, or control my emotions. I felt like I was on an unending rollercoaster ride with my heart and mind racing uncontrollably. Fortunately, my background in stress management helped me to cope with the ups and downs. Years of medical and educational knowledge also helped me to self-advocate.

I was grateful for family and friends who supported me through this transformational period of time. My son was even able to take leave from the Navy to be at my side. It was time for me to take a step back, learn acceptance, and allow myself to graciously receive from others. Until now, my whole life had been about control and giving to others, especially as a corporate manager and educator.

My daughter brought in plant-based supplements, organic protein drinks, and peanut butter with coconut, fresh water from a nearby artesian spring, a diffuser with Young Living oils, my cold laser light, fresh flowers, crystals, healing music, and even window sun catchers to brighten my room. My family then teamed together to prepare my home's bedroom with a hospital bed and made space for me to move around with a wheelchair or walker when I returned home. It was a miracle to have a medical equipment provider in the area to lend them the bed and needed medical supplies without cost. My children even freshly painted my bedroom walls, cleared any clutter, and replaced the flooring to create a clean and comfortable spiritual/healing sanctuary.

It was a long 30 days to get my scarred lungs to bring more oxygen into the blood stream to support better circulation and movement. I began transitioning from the wheelchair to using a walker for short distances. As my energy began returning, I cheered on the older residents within the facility to support and inspire them in their own healing processes. Nurses joined me in my healing sanctuary during breaks to escape stresses of their busy day and allow time to chat. Love overflowed from my heart as I was surrounded by others, quickly learning the importance of divine love and acceptance.

About three months after returning home, the "voice" visited me to inform me it was important to wean off medications within six months. As my intuition had grown significantly during my healing process, I knew my body was suffering and began to experience even more side effects. Having learned to listen to my inner self, I began developing a wellness team to assist me in the next segment of my journey. This journey taught me to believe in myself, choosing to trust, have faith, and accept divine love. Although doctors advised against ending the medications, I chose to trust my inner guidance.

Combining my experiences as a stress management specialist, working with energy healing techniques and my knowledge of the medical field, I began to slowly and carefully wean myself off the medications. My wellness team consisted of a nephrologist, cardiologist, integrative medical doctor, acupuncturist, multi-modality chiropractor, physical therapist, cranial-sacral therapist, massage therapist, yoga instructor, and numerous energy workers. They worked in unity to assist and support my healing process.

Although there is a time and place for medications, I knew my body needed to detox from the steroids and chemo drugs. One of the key components to healing from the inside out included a plant-based nutritional diet and supplement plan to reinforce the healing transformation. My diet consisted of at least five helpings of protein each day and an abundant amount of organic fruits, vegetables, and herbs. My body was highly sensitive to chlorine, so pure water was critical. My children brought me fresh water from the spring to avoid further toxins. Soon the side-effects began to disappear. As written in my first published educational book, *Project Reality*, "It takes a community to educate a child," and I believe it also takes a caring community to heal oneself from dis-ease.

Life is a journey infused with lessons from our failures,

mistakes and/or sufferings. This experience with lupus taught me to go within to unite with my true self and surrender to God when I felt weak and alone. Never before had I allowed myself to truly receive loving, compassionate care from others and connect to God/Source/Universe so closely.

The truth is there is no reason to face our struggles alone for we are never truly alone. Instead, step out and know with all of your heart how deeply loved you are just as you are. Even in the emptiest of moments, we always have a CHOICE in how we perceive a situation at hand. I chose life and learned forgiveness, acceptance, gratitude and love. I now seek out the positives in all that occurs in my life.

My body no longer allowed me to rush forward in anything. Everything I did was a step by step process, including relearning how to breathe, walk, and move. Instead of treating life as a race and rushing through it to the end, my body demanded a slower pace and more patience. It was time to learn a deeper level of self-love. This next level of healing included forgiving from my childhood and integrating with my inner child. In addition, meditation and breathing exercises eliminated the mind chatter and allowed for stillness to open doors to new possibilities.

Despite struggling through lupus, I have been inspired by my dis-ease to embrace life and share my story of miracles as an author and speaker. To enhance my current education and knowledge after hours of webinars, online trainings, and personal coaching, I have also committed to completing a doctorate in integrative health. The many teachings enhance the resilience of the body, mind, and spirit. Our bodies are resilient and continuously rebuild when we practice self-love through regular self-care of chemical-free hydration and nutrition, along with movement and self-compassion. I now pay close attention to my environment, what I put in my mouth, emotional upsets, thoughts and the voice within that guides me.

Each morning, I start my day with gratitude that I am alive and for the miracle of life I was gifted. Feeling very blessed, I do my best to make the most of each day. It is an important discovery to become more conscious and aware of one's thoughts, emotions, actions, habits and old belief systems to strengthen the healing process.

Life is a process of giving and receiving. After receiving much care and support from others, I am ready to share what I have learned. This enables me to touch other's lives and provide hope and inspiration. Like the metamorphosis of a caterpillar into a butterfly, I am ready to come out of my healing cocoon. The time has arrived to support others in attaining their own miraculous health and joy-filled lives.

In love and compassion, my purpose is to inspire hope and be a living example that miracles are possible. By following my truths, and honoring who I am, unlimited miracles, that lay within, are revealed. To live, change was inevitable. Integrating the unity of mind, body, and spirit, my life will be forever different. Like the caterpillar, it's often in the midst of struggling through change that we discover the wings we never knew we had.

About the Author

Diane McKee

2020 brings in an opportunity to wake up miracles and establish new beginnings for the next decade. As I look back, I have experienced many miracles throughout my life, and I am grateful for each experience. I have learned that "Life is a choice, and anything is possible if I allow miracles to happen." Through my experiences, I have learned to find positives in every situation, good or bad. I have chosen LIFE and wish to share what I have learned throughout my journey. I chose to provide hope and inspiration as I move forward. If you are open and ready to receive, I am available to assist, educate, or just provide hope and inspiration with auto-immune challenges or other life-shattering circumstances. Through my experiences, I found that it is not enough to only work with one's physical self, but to Wake-Up Miracles, it requires working with the mind, emotions, and spirit as well.

My passion continues to be absorbing knowledge as a student of life and sharing knowledge in the areas of health care and education. I enjoy music, working with children, pets and the elderly while working with the love and appreciation of Mother Earth through master gardening.

My skills and abilities include business ownership of Pathways to Relaxation, now renamed to Pathways to Miracles. I have become a biofeedback specialist, transformational coach, Reiki master teacher, yoga teacher, reflexologist, numerologist and educational teacher graduating Magna Cum Laude with a B.S. in Elementary and Physical Education, working towards becoming an international self-help author and speaker. I have trained with talented individuals from Mind Valley Institute, Native Americans, shamans, Mayan priests, a Tibetan miracle healer, along with many others to enhance my skills. I am currently a student at Quantum University working towards my Doctorate in Integrative Medicine. This learning provides an incredible amount of information from my instructors in the areas of nutrition, autoimmune, brain health, anti-aging techniques, and more.

My background and experiences include:

- Stress management business incorporating many of the skill-sets listed above
- Work with clients for a decade, administrating biofeedback sessions, teaching stress reduction and yoga, and performing reflexology
- FedEx Corporate management for over 10 years with two years in senior management
- Experiencing loss of a child with a nongenetic heart defect and the birth of three other children
- Licensed elementary and physical education teaching experiences
- CNA/ward clerk experiences in a nursing home, doctors' offices, and ER
- Raised on a 300+acre dairy farm enjoying nature and learning strong morals and work ethics.

It is not meant for my knowledge to stay within me, but to share it with others. My wish is to be a part of your health team to enhance quality of life for you, your children, and generations to come. Below is my listed contact information to connect with my coaching and speaking gifts. Allow yourself to wake up and start your transformational journey to new beginnings and miracles.

Contact Information:

Email: PathwaysToMiracles@yahoo.com
Text Messaging, Requests for appointments only please: 262-349-0585

At this time, I offer telephone appointments only. Please contact me by email or text messaging as found above, to set up your free 30-minute telephone consultation. My intention is to work with new clients as a guiding light, providing inspiration and hope as we work together in Waking-Up Miracles. Anything is possible if you allow miracles to happen.

CHANGING LIFE IN ARUBA

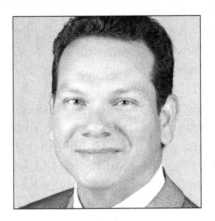

Dr. Sandy Roga

U pon graduation in March 2003, I was eager to start working and making a difference in people's lives. It did not take long for this to occur and continue throughout my career. One day, two parents showed up with long faces and were very desperate. During the consultation, they told me that their baby girl had not slept since she was born and was two months old at the time. She had been crying nonstop. The only time she was quiet for a few minutes was when she was breastfeeding. They had been to their general physician, pediatrician, and midwife with no change, since they did not know what was happening to the baby.

When I examined the baby, she was crying in a Moro reflex posture. It was like she was telling me that she had a terrible headache, and no one has been able to understand her. Her vitals appeared to be normal with a slight increase of her heart rate. While examining her spine, a significant subluxation was noted at her atlas. It was literally displaced to the left and posterior. As a chiropractor in Aruba, I was not allowed to take X-rays and was not about to expose this little baby to radiation for something that was easy to find. I explained in detail to the parents what I was going to do to correct her subluxation. I placed my activator on the left atlas and adjusted her and then gently placed my pinky fingers on her atlas.

Within 20 seconds of making the correction, she turned her head around and smiled at me, stopped crying, and went to sleep. I told her parents to let her sleep because she needed to recover for the time, she remained awake for so long. Also, it was important to breastfeed her while she slept. I recommended the parents bring her in the next day to see how she was doing. When they arrived the following day with their baby, the parents had smiles on their faces, looked well-rested, and had a lot of questions. Their baby girl had slept 16 hours straight, which made them concerned at a given point because they did not know that she would sleep for that long. And when she woke up, she wasn't crying anymore and had a beautiful smile on her face. When the parents handed me their child, I became very emotional while holding the baby in my arms because I knew that I had made a significant change in this child's life and future. She looked at me straight in the eyes with a big smile and it felt like she was thanking me for helping her.

Mrs. Lourdes' Story

The daughter of my patient came in very concerned about her mother because she had a stomach condition that was not improving. I told her to convince her mom to come in so I could discuss her condition. Finally, the mother decided to come in with a letter from her socialized insurance saying that she had a neck pain that would not go away. Immediately, I noticed she was not doing well, that she had lost a lot of weight, and she had a yellowish skin tone. I asked her to tell me what she was feeling because it was clear that it was more than just neck pain. She was also very stressed and disappointed because she was recently diagnosed with stomach cancer. When she had her first chemotherapy session, she almost died. Her oncologist told her immediately to discontinue treatment because it would kill her before the cancer did.

Wake Up: Miracles

She continued explaining what she was feeling by telling me that she had been having diarrhea for months and anything she ate would not stay down. The diarrhea was accompanied by constant pain and since she wasn't digesting anything, she was losing a lot of weight. She struggled to even drink water. Her oncologist did not advise her of anything else that she could do to help her condition. I told her that I couldn't treat the cancer but what I could do is help improve her health by making a lot of changes and helping to stop her autoimmune response. Her body created the cancer and if the body is given the chance, it will get rid of the cancer.

With the help of her two daughters, I spent a lot of time explaining lifestyle changes that would improve her health. Her diet was also changed with the specific use of home remedies. A specific care plan was made for her at the clinic to decrease her stress, to let her sleep so she could recover, and stop her sympathetic response. The care plan also consisted of improving her immune response to give her a fighting chance. Her energy was improved with multiple devices and she was advised to spend a lot of time in nature while grounding her body. Detox programs were implemented to get rid of any possible toxins she might have in her body.

Not much occurred during the first three months, but she was finally able to digest a little food and was able to keep water down. Then, specific supplements were introduced to her diet after absorption was improved. The main point of adjustment because the vagus nerve and rehabilitating it to provide her with proper vagal tone. Together, a great fight was given to her and great results started to show. Adjustments continued weekly for the next six months. Slowly, she started to reach proper hydration and digest food. Her diarrhea began to subside, and she started to regain weight. Her skin color improved from a yellowish-white color to a more vibrant tone. Decreased stress improved her mood and allowed her to express herself with a more positive and assertive attitude. This patient's stomach pain had decreased, and she was able to enjoy meals without being scared of what would happen next.

She is currently enjoying life again with no traces of the

stomach cancer. This patient is still under my care and being advised on her lifestyle changes that she has to maintain, staying with the proper attitude for life. This woman is a fighter and was given a fair chance to fight for her health.

Zaydee's Story

A three-year-old girl was brought to me with the inability to walk, talk, or express herself. At 11 months, she contracted chicken pox and immediately went from a normal child to being unable to sit or even hold her head up. She was also having digestive problems with an inability to eat properly. She was sent to her pediatrician, then the neurologist, then to Colombia for more opinions. When they came back to Aruba, her parents were told that everything seemed to be normal and nothing else could be done to help her. Her mother was not about to give up on Zaydee, especially since she was told that her child would have to live with her deficiency for the rest of her life. After the initial exam, I told the mother that we were going to adjust Zaydee to see if we could wake up her brain and see what happens. It would be a long-term care plan; no promises were given because nobody knew exactly how she would react.

Together with my colleague who was an osteopath, we designed a care plan for Zaydee. Her adjustment consisted of cranial, spinal, and visceral adjustments. Immediately after the initial adjustments, we started to notice changes with Zaydee. I became very excited for this result because this proved to us with the hope that her brain function could improve. As we continued to adjust her, something new would show up each time. She made her first attempt to walk and started to say her first words. Each time something happened, our emotions were getting higher and higher due to the exit results.

After one year of adjustments, a girl who was told that she would never walk had started to walk on her own. She walked in the office and hugged me so hard that my eyes had tears of joy. Then the words started coming out of her mouth—not clearly, but she started to express her feelings. Zaydee was able to become independent and help herself. Her language has improved significantly even though she was unable to say all the words clearly, but she was now able to communicate with her family and friends. Her digestive system improved, leading to a normal appetite and rapid, normal growth. Even though she has not reached her full potential yet, Zaydee went from a girl who struggled with walking, talking, and unable to properly processing information and expressing herself to doing all these essential skills to help herself in this world.

Michael's Story

Michael came in on his first visit with complaints of neck pain due to intense stress. He was in IT and spent a lot of time at a computer, with lots of pressure to perform. He also complained of chest pain and difficulty breathing, with an intense pain through his entire left arm. He had all the signs of having a heart attack. Immediately, I started to check his vitals and told my staff to call 911. I continued to lay him down and he went into shock. His entire body started to shake and tremble, and he was having trouble talking to me and breathing. Michael started to sweat profusely. To calm him down, I started to do a cranial release technique and then went to adjust his C1 gently and rehab his cranial nerve using quantum neurology. It seemed like forever, but it had taken the ambulance almost 15 minutes to arrive.

By the time they arrived, his breathing had improved, his chest pain had started to normalize, and his neck and arm pain had decreased. Michael was still shaking a little and was cold due to the profuse sweating. I told the EMT how he came in and what I had done to help. They immediately checked his vitals and did an ECG on him to see how he was doing. He was much better but went into hysteria while the EMTs were evaluating him, so they decided to take him to the hospital to do further testing and keep him under observation.

The following day, Michael showed up at the clinic, walking in with a huge smile on his face like nothing had happened. The doctors said that he was lucky because he was having a heart attack but could not explain how the process was stopped. When the ambulance reached the hospital, all he wanted to do was sleep, and that is what he did. He woke up feeling great the next day and they released him from the hospital. Since then, he has been under my care and never had a similar episode, even though he is still in IT at this time with his own business and different types of stress.

Aunty Chichi's Story

I woke up feeling very sick with the flu. I was about to decide not going to work, but something inside of me said to go and keep on helping as many people as I could. During the morning my cousin Mario called my wife with an emergency. My Aunty Chichi's blood pressure had suddenly dropped and she was not recovering from it. The general physician told Mario to call the family to say goodbye because she was dying. My wife Jeanine told Mario to bring her in immediately to see what I could do for her.

When they arrived, my aunty was so weak and disoriented that she did not even recognize when she was being wheeled in. I used two adjustment techniques on her. First, I gently applied the Arthrostim to her C1 after carefully using KST occipital drop to ask where to adjust. Then I proceeded to do a cranial release technique (CRT) and applied a quantum neurology light called GRT to the base of her skull during the adjustment. I told my CA's to put her on the PEMF for 45 minutes with a GRT light at the base of her skull and told them to keep her under constant supervision and that I would reassess her when she was done with the PEMF.

After I came out of one of my adjusting rooms, I saw my aunt stand up on her own and walk out of the healing room without assistance. When she saw me, she actually recognized me and said, "Hi, Sandy," and walked out of the office like nothing had been wrong. The patient in the office who saw her enter in a wheelchair disoriented, confused, and dying could not believe what had just happened. I had tears of joy because I saw my aunty alive again. I immediately remembered how powerful chiropractic is and I continued to adjust more people that day with a renewed energy and passion.

The next day she came back because I did not get the chance to talk to her and reassess her properly. The first thing she did was to give me a big hug and thanked me for giving her the energy to live again.

My aunt is now 87 years old and still alive three years after her family was told that she was dying. The thing is I woke up sick that day and wasn't planning on coming to work, but God and the Universe had a different plan for me. From that point on, it became very clear to me that I have to use my intuition every time I get a message and not to be afraid to manifest the information being sent to me.

About the Author

Dr. Sandy Roga, DC

Sandy was born and raised in Aruba and left to play baseball and get an education in the United States when he was 19. During his senior year playing baseball at Cumberland University while icing a left shoulder in the training room, a chiropractor showed up to work with the football players. The chiropractor asked him what the problem was and then asked if he could work with Sandy. After the adjustment, Sandy felt a difference. The next day when he went to throw a baseball, Sandy did not feel the sharp pain in his shoulder and immediately decided to become a chiropractor.

He graduated in March 2003 as a Doctor of Chiropractic and he has been working for 17 years in his practice, Quality Chiropractic Clinic, in Aruba. Sandy has also coached baseball for 17 years and was the President of the Olympic Medical Committee of Aruba for 15 years. He has been married to Jeanine Roga-Wernet for 16 years and has two beautiful children, Scarlet (11) and Jean Paul (8).

Contact Information:

Quality Chiropractic Clinic
Primavera 6-J, Wayaka
Aruba
Phone: (297) 588-5487 / Cell: (297) 592-6625
Email: chirogaruba@hotmail.com

THE DYING ORPHAN IN INDIA

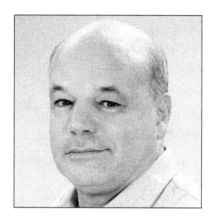

Ed Strachar

Working as a remote spiritual healer brings many interesting cases. Remote, means that I work at any distance, usually through the internet or phone to anyone around the world. Healing means to be made whole. Cure, in effect; not just treat or suppress symptoms, but go direct to the cause.

Since everything is energy, all starts at the energetic level. What controls energy is the intelligence field that forms the energy into something functional. That is what we call a spirit. Once we say the word spirit, it triggers many reactions, religious connotations, etc. yet keeping it simple, and fundamentally scientific, the word "spirit" merely forms the energy into something functional. Being a spiritual healer, I work at this energy and spiritual level or what some call "metaphysical" level that few can see, many question and some doubt it even exists altogether. Metaphysical simply means beyond the physical level. It's not visible with the naked eye, so some don't believe it exists.

As I was about to head out of my office about 10 p.m. one evening, I received a desperate message from Thambi Mulupuri, the founder of an orphanage named Thambi's Kids Home in Eluru, India. I have sponsored Thambi's home for many years and many friends have gone to see him and donate their time and love for the children. Thambi had messaged that evening, telling me that one of his children, Ramya, an Indian girl about 9-10 years old, was desperately sick. Her life force was fading before everyone's eyes. Poor and desperate, he brought her to the hospital using the last funds he had, funds reserved for food for the children, in a desperate attempt to save her life.

The doctors told him that her blood platelet count was going down drastically, to a near fatal level. They gave her medicine at considerable expense, yet her condition simply got worse. He asked if I could help. Having to google what blood platelets actually were, so I had a basic understanding, *platelets, as I learned*, are the tiny *blood* cells that help your body form clots to stop bleeding. If one of your *blood* vessels is damaged, it sends out signals to the *platelets. The platelets* then rush to the site and form a plug (clot) to fix the damage. [www.urmc.rochester.edu/encyclopedia/]

What I could see at the spiritual level was that the child's life force was dangerously low at 45% and had a severe and heavy dark energy on her. I knew what I had to do.

The child was in the orphanage, having returned from the hospital, lying limp looking ready to die. I performed a short healing session with Thambi through online chat, as I usually do with him. Although I was across the ocean at the time, physical distance is immaterial when working at higher dimensions of energy, and in this case, the dimensions of the soul, which is beyond space and time. I removed the heavy, dark energy, something that took me 20 years to develop the power/ability to do, and then restored her life force/soul. Since I had never met the girl, I had to work through Thambi whom I had a strong connection with, to make sure I had a solid soul path of love to the child.

I then energized a bottle of water he held in his hands for her. As Thambi reported, she started waking up and was given the water. I left, and the session ended. Within 20 minutes, Thambi messaged me back fervently, she seemed alive and well again, he stated! Thambi rushed her to the hospital again for a blood platelet count and was thunderstruck. Her platelets had returned to the upper of edge of what was normal, and the child had recovered completely. Several years later, as I tell this story, she has been continuously healthy.

Few understand the power of darkness and the negative effects it can have on someone. As Nikola Tesla once said:

"The day science begins to study non-physical phenomena, it will make more progress in one decade than in all the previous centuries of its existence."

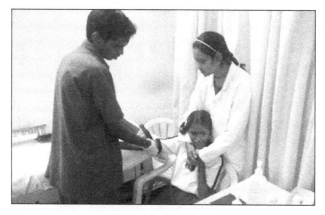

Ramya in the Hospital

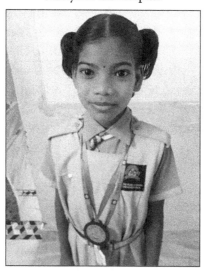

Ramya after, October 2019

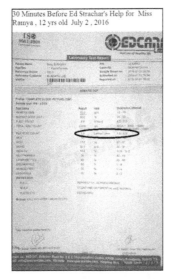
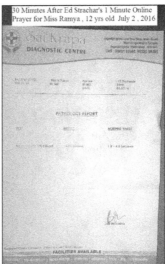

Platelet count increased from 1.0 to 4.5 [Normal rage: 1.5—4.5]

About the Author

Ed Strachar

Ed Strachar is an Elite Healer, one of the planet's most powerful, with many medically validated cases of healing remotely strictly through online chat and phone. Documented cases that involved life threatening diseases such as Stage IV cancer, Tuberculosis, Crohn's disease, and has a 90+% success rate with depression, anxiety, high blood pressure, atrial fibrillations, and also orthopedic issues such as bad knees, hips, shoulders and other joints, saving numerous clients from joint replacement surgery.

Many refer to him as a miracle worker, yet he quickly points out that this is a learnable skill and not based on religion, faith, or miracles.

Strachar has learned to access soul-restoring life force energy from very high dimensions. A nonreligious approach using advanced energy medicine, vibrational healing, and spiritual science principles. Many medical doctors, naturopaths, nurses and the like now rely on his advice and abilities.

He is the author of the upcoming book, *Magical Energy, Miracle Healing*.

Contact Information:

If you would like to learn more, please visit
www.HealingGenius.com or
www.facebook.com/EdStracharSpiritHealer

FROM DEVASTATION TO RESTORATION, THE BRAIN CAN RESET ITSELF

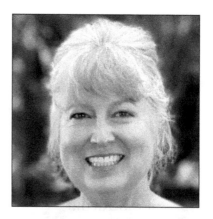

Rhonda Grillo

L ife is so unpredictable. Who knew I would become an emergency "student" in the brain wellness industry? This particular curve life threw at me was something I sure didn't see coming. However, looking back on my life makes me realize that it is the substantial surprises that potentially can become blessings in which we touch the lives of others and hopefully leave the world a better place.

My story begins with my 23-year-old daughter who was injured while skiing. After falling and hitting the back of her head, she was diagnosed with a traumatic brain injury (TBI). The TBI diagnosis immediately commanded my full and focused attention! Even the words "traumatic brain injury" sound so scary and devastating. My journey into the world of brain injury, trauma, rehabilitation, and restoration began, and this educational journey has been one of the scariest and fascinating trips I've ever taken.

My background of working as a private flight instructor and employment with a major airline did not prepare me for this fascinating adventure into the inner workings of the brain. However, being a lifelong learner, truth seeker and myth buster since childhood did prepare me for my search for truth and healing. As a result, this new and unexplored territory caused me to immediately immerse myself into learning all the information possible on the brain.

Can you imagine my panic when receiving the call that my daughter was in and out of consciousness as a result of her head injury? My imagination was filled with fear as I considered all of the worst-case scenarios. Questions rampaged inside my conscious brain. Would she be able to recover and live a normal life? Would she be able to function at work or even maintain a job? Would she be able to enjoy personal relationships? As her mother, my feelings were that her future, known or unknown, rested in my ability to ferret out the best path to her full recovery. My passion for helping her heal propelled me into action. But where should I start? Even though she was 23 years old at the time of her injury, she was still my baby and her healing became my number one priority.

Several years before "the accident" my daughter had been a passionate high school volleyball player, always contributing 100% effort and as a result, experienced a few concussions. She was the best when it came to playing her part on the team and coaches loved her for it. Being super competitive, if it was physically possible, she hit the ball skillfully and on target whether it meant a drop and roll or literally diving and sliding on the ground to get the hit. Constant bruises were her companions but knowing she always gave it her best shot was satisfying to her. The accumulative effect of several blows to the head can be devastating and it certainly was for her. It was back then that I started researching concussions and the effect on the brain.

Now my new research began investigating the long-term impact of repeated concussions to the brain. These concussions had caused her to have severe sleep issues and gradually she developed adrenal fatigue, impacting her health in several ways and zapping her energy. As if that wasn't enough, when she was a high school junior, she ended up with mono and had to quit playing volleyball. This devastated her. She became very depressed and we sought help with different modalities that didn't seem to be very effective. Remembering this experience, I knew that most of the traditional brain treatments we had already tried such as biofeedback and neurofeedback hadn't helped her, so I had to find something that would.

It is important to note that my daughter was rigid about eating healthy, exercising, and maintaining optimal health to perform at the highest level. Driven toward success, her ambitious, diligent, and committed efforts allowed her to excel academically and physically. Her joy and happiness with life was contagious and I never worried about her ability to succeed. What a joy it was to watch her be a star on her team and achieve success in so many areas of her life. She was very entertaining to watch play and a surge to my 'Mama pride.' She was going far in life and I wouldn't need to worry about her.

However, after the TBI my daughter changed drastically. After a great deal of praying for guidance for her healing, I found our first well-known brain clinic, which specialized in TBI-type injuries. They offered the gamut of possibilities and were quite popular with football players and other high-profile patients with brain injuries. Cost was not an issue; the money would be found somehow, someway. My quest for help with her healing became unstoppable.

After spending thousands of dollars and dozens of hours at the clinic, unfortunately my daughter still suffered from severe depression, anxiety, hopelessness, despair, fearfulness and apathy among other symptoms. Unable to help, the next suggestion from the doctor was to start medicating her with antidepressants and anti-anxiety pills. Heavy medication was not seriously considered for my once vivacious and active child; doping her on pills seemed extremely counter-intuitive. There had to be a healthier, prudent, and more natural way to help her. I really wanted to find a noninvasive, proven, and safe way to help her brain help itself. This would be ideal.

There are different levels of injury to the brain, and fortunately hers was not the "worst" compared to so many others with significant TBI. Having just started working on her first job as an auditor with a major company, then losing the job post-injury compounded her challenges with a new lack of confidence and isolation. A further worry emerged two months post-injury when she shared that she had lost her faith in God, even questioning whether God existed. Her declaration was quite shocking since pre-injury her faith was unshakeable. Something was very wrong inside her brain; the daughter we knew was slipping away. A further indicator of her abject trauma came during a mother-daughter trip to Austria and Switzerland to hike the Alps several months after her TBI. This trip ended in the discovery that her once great passion for travel had vanished. Reflecting on our before-daughter to our after-daughter, my husband and I realized that several aspects of her personality traits, beliefs, and behaviors had changed drastically.

Her lack of motivation was the most disconcerting. She went from one extreme to another, from super ambitious to low motivation that caused us much concern. What if she couldn't go back to work? What if we had to take care of her the rest of our lives? Would she ever get back to "normal" again? With an unknown future glaring at us and a fragile, injured, and anxiety-ridden daughter facing such a mysterious abyss, we carefully journeyed forward, talking to people, sharing our story, searching for better answers, and seeking better treatments. So far, nothing had really made a difference in her healing process and I wondered if anything ever would.

Truly, there is a natural flow to life's journey of discovering the truth, the answers and the wisdom sought comes if we continue to seek knowledge and notice the opportunities presented to us instead of wallowing in the negative aspects of the situation. Where there is life, there is always hope. Never giving up or giving in to the fear and worry, God led me to the discovery of how to help our dear daughter.

After church service one Sunday morning, a shy man who doesn't ordinarily stay around to chat told me an intriguing story about his wife's niece who hadn't been able to attend high school anymore because of several concussions from playing basketball.

She had reached the point that she couldn't perform math exercises nor comprehend her reading and had even lost her ability to play the piano. She'd suffered more than most people and the family had tried all Western and Eastern brain therapies and medicine they could find, seeking help. Unfortunately, nothing made a noticeable difference. My mom "antennas" perked right up; the next day my daughter and I were on the phone talking with her and her mom about their journey to wellness.

When she found the technology that helped her, she had reached the point of despair and initially wasn't willing to try it. After all, she'd tried everything else to no avail, so why face disappointment of another treatment failing to provide any improvement and then suffering the subsequent hopelessness?

Finally, after several months of stalling, this young lady decided to move forward. It took about six months of applications for her brain to fully relax, rebalance, and reset itself into a more optimized and reliable "captain of the plane" again. Just like the body can heal a cut, the brain has the innate ability to regenerate itself into wellness and rehabilitate itself into a trustworthy and dependable control center, as a result of neuroplasticity.[1] This is the innate function of the brain to create and reorganize synaptic connections, especially in response to cognitive development post injury. She regained not only her brain functions, but she also returned to school and continued on to college. She is now happily married. An awesome end to what could have been a never-ending tragedy.

Inspired by this story, my daughter started the process of this technology immediately and continues using them to this day.

Although assisting the brain's innate ability to relax, rebalance, and reset took several months, slowly my daughter began to return to her "normal" pre-injury self. Natural healing modalities take a lot longer to notice a difference if compared to the instant gratification of medications, but the journey is worth it. After getting her faith back, her depression and anxiety improved, and my daughter became more confident and less fearful. It was a six-month journey before she was able to work again and gain her motivation back. Now we had our own proof that brains can rewire and heal themselves.[2]

After a year and a half of living with us and regaining her confidence, she moved to another state and has been able to cope with and respond to stress resiliently. Her symptoms are gone. She works online, supports herself financially, and is very thankful for her restored brain wellness. She plans on moving to a foreign country this year to fulfill her dream of living abroad.

I'm now madly in love with the study of our brain. Seriously. So complex, infinite, and magnificent, yet so very delicate and frail; our brain is the pilot of the plane. It controls the body, mind, and spirit. A healthy brain is the foundation to overall health, happiness, and everything in between. Without it being in balance, the body can't function properly, the mind is confused or distraught, and all sorts of discomfort emerge including disease.[3] It's a complex problem that exhausts the mind and then the body. An out-of-balance brain is equivalent to four flat tires on the plane but expecting the pilot to be able to take off risk free. Not happening! If you're going to get to your desired destination, something's got to change.

The sad part is that most people accept the flat tires and live their lives in what I call "survival mode," which becomes the new norm, instead of thriving as we were meant to. Our brains and bodies do workarounds so that we can keep surviving.

A wholesome captain makes solid choices, wise decisions, and flies safe. The goal of this brain mirroring technology is to provide your brain with the truths it needs to repair and rewire itself. The sessions are NOT EMDR, hyperbaric oxygen, or any of the other most commonly known therapies that retrain, force, or direct the brain. Many of those therapies we had tried in the past and dismissed as ineffective several years before when she'd suffered from the concussions.

Wouldn't you trust in the brain's own innate wisdom to rewire itself rather than someone forcing it to do what they think is best? This technology gives our clients confidence and allows them to trust the process because they have everything to gain and nothing to lose from this proven, noninvasive, and completely safe process.

After my daughter's recovery, I personally started using this modality because I had only snoozed at night but not slept for over 30 years due to chronic pain and stress. After just a few in-office sessions, I started dreaming again and sleeping deeply for seven or more hours. My disease ravaged body started healing and restoring itself for the first time in years and my energy returned. This too, was a miracle. I was so inspired by our experience and its impact on our lives that I became a business owner, incorporating this miraculous technology to help others regain their health and overcome stress, improve energy and mood stability, and enjoy deep, quality sleep.

Whether someone has suffered from an injury or just wants a healthier and sharper brain, everyone can enjoy major improvements in brain function including potentially improving cognition skills including memory, focus, learning, and problem solving. The brain is an infinite possibility; exploration precedes discovery and the risk you take is often worth it. The personal success stories of those who have experienced this technology are so gratifying.

Who knew that a 94-year-old man stuck in grief and loneliness from his wife's death could become balanced and dwell in joy, peace, and regain his desire to live? A wonderful addition to his story is that his memory was restored from a debilitating memory loss disease and he is now able to read books and do crossword puzzles for the first time in many years.

Further, who knew that a 54-year-old man would not only get the best quality sleep of his entire life after being a light sleeper, but also gain improved vision, lose his car sickness, and his claustrophobia? And, what a gift it was when his lost memory of his childhood returned after just three of these mirroring sessions.

And further, an attorney who just wanted to be sharper in the courtroom through faster memorization of jurors' names and quicker, more reliable recall, would do exactly that.

These are just a small sampling of the amazing discoveries of my clients who came to my office after I learned how to help people receive the wondrous help my daughter obtained after her struggle to return to thriving instead of just surviving her life. This year has been the busiest yet the most satisfying year of my life. Four years ago I would have never had the energy or brain power to be successful in business, yet alone even work full-time. Now I'm blessed with the ability to assist many people on their journey to wellness through optimized brain function resulting in restored hope, happiness, and well being.

One client said, "You owe it to yourself (and your brain) to see the many ways your life can be improved through an optimized brain." I agree. To begin the process of your miracle story, contact me for more information about this cutting-edge technology that helped my daughter, myself, and so many others start thriving again.

[1] www.gemmlearning.com/blog/learning_science/how-neuroplasticity-was-discovered/

[2] Andrew Zaleski, *The Power of Neuroplasticity: Boy's Brain Rewires Itself Even With 1/6th of Its Contents Missing*, Sott.net: One Zero, Feb. 27, 2019. https://sott.net/en408390

[3] Daniel Mate, M.D., *When the Body Says No* (John Wiley & Sons, Inc., 2003)

About the Author

Rhonda Grillo

Rhonda is enjoying her 30th year of marriage with her wonderful husband, Galen,and is the mother of three adult children who are her pride and joy, Early in life she earned her commercial pilot license and flight instructor certificate. In addition, she enjoyed a 25-year career with a major airline before taking early retirement in 2008.

Following her daughter's traumatic brain injury in February 2017, she became a student of the brain to help her during the long journey to recovery.. She currently enjoys helping others optimize their brain, whether they've had trauma or not, so they too can thrive instead of just survive their lives.

Contact Information:

For a complimentary consultation you may email her: HealyMeNow@gmail.com or call (866) HEALYME (432-5963)

THE MIRACLE OF BEING IN PRACTICE

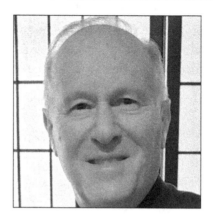

Dr. Dennis Harper

Miracle, a noun meaning "amazing or wonderful occurrence," comes from the Latin *miraculum,* "object of wonder." Dig way back and the word derives from *smeiros,* meaning, "to smile," which is exactly what you do when a miracle happens. To quote the American French author Anais Nin, "The dream was always running ahead of me. To catch up, to live for a moment in unison with it, that was the miracle." Just ask any rock star.

We all have definitions in life of what a miracle means. It is different for everybody. With that said I get to make up my own miracles. About 20 years ago I had a consultant ask me to write up all the things that happened to make me the person I am today. I started out "I was born November 9, 1956 in Crescent City California," a small town of 2,500 people. That was the start of my miracle.

We tend to find the things that define us, and our purpose in life. We should view every day as a miracle. I go to bed every night saying, "This was the best day of my life," and in the morning I look in the mirror and say, "This is going to be the best day of my life." Looking back at the miracles of the last 64 years and finding defining moments makes me the special person I am that makes me a miracle!

My memories of kindergarten and first grade helped define the direction of my life. Without realizing it, that allowed me to discover many miracles. It directed me on a pathway to change the world.

Kindergarten and The Little Girl

I started kindergarten at 4 1/2 years old. My family thought it was okay for me to go to school early. My parents felt that having an education was extremely important, so they put me in a Catholic school starting in the first grade. The Catholic school was strict. I wore a gray tie, red shirt, with salt-and-pepper corduroy pants. I remember the first time doing the Pledge of Allegiance out in front of the school.

The first and second grades were in the same room together; third/fourth, fifth/six, seventh/eighth were grouped accordingly. There were about 18 students per classroom. Things that stood out to me were: When I went into the first grade, I ended up sitting on the second-grade side for the first two weeks and nobody caught it. I was five years old. When it was finally discovered, I was told I was wrong, and Sister Bosco hollered at me and made me get back on my side of the room. I had no idea where I was supposed to be.

Sister B.... came to my desk, opened it up, said it was a mess, and took everything out and threw it on the floor. I peed my pants. It was one of the most traumatic things to me. I was very embarrassed.

After being relocated in the room I sat across from a beautiful little girl. Time has erased her name. She sat in the next row by a tall, narrow window. This girl had beautiful blonde hair that would sparkle in the sunlight. She was gone a lot from school and I never understood why. My memory of her was about March of 1962. I remember this was Easter time and I had gotten her a little teddy bear. She was dead a month later of leukemia. Being five years old, I didn't really know what that meant. There was no grief counseling or any of that back then.

In the third and fourth grade, I would sit and draw pictures and gaze out the window. I would draw people walking in circles of radio waves to heal them of things. I am not sure where the ideas came from. There was no Internet or news that talked about healing with radio waves in the '60s. Looking back you have to wonder what is guiding you. Where do those ideas come from? How do they get there? What drives you to make them happen? Thoughts of the "little blond girl" sat in the depths of my brain until about four years ago. I had not thought about it or the reasons I had been driven in all those years. Was it the little blonde girl that drove me to learn how to heal people?

My goal when I started my practice was to get in, start three practices, get rich, and get out. I was 20 when I started Chiropractic College; I had just turned 21 and graduated at 23 with my Doctor of Chiropractic degree. I had a real drive to start a practice. However, I went broke with the first practice I was in. I took a bunch of consulting courses, did different things, started back again, started making money, and started investing it. Everything I invested in; I lost money. It did not matter if it was real estate, stocks and bonds, trading futures—whatever I did, it seemed like nothing worked.

My practice was doing well; I was traveling and putting together my own training program. I was pushing all the time, running between the practice and trainings. Later I learned that my staff were concerned that I was headed for a nervous breakdown. At that time, I reached a point in my marriage where I had tried everything I could to make it work, yet I was not happy. We were living together yet we weren't connected in any other way. I realized I was drinking too much in an attempt to numb myself, and I had to get out. A woman I knew helped open the door to learning what my feelings really were. In that imagery, the picture of the little girl came up. In my brain I cried for two weeks. It was like, "Oh my gosh, that's why everything I've done to this point in time has not been successful, because I had a different purpose in life."

Recognizing my purpose allowed me to make better choices. When I started making those choices with the idea of changing the world, all those doors began to open up. My teaching has improved, my presentations became better. The people I meet in my life have become a greater source of joy. Every day is the best day of my life since then and the next day is better yet. It's amazing; every incident seems to build on the next and more ideas come into my brain all the time. Depending on who you talk to, we know/assume/believe that all the ideas in the world are in the Universe if your mind is open to hear them. Whether you believe in "God" or in a god, or the energy of the Universe, if you allow yourself to be open you can hear and feel almost everything that happens.

The story of the little girl; was it an emotional driver? Or was it an experience? It could have been either, or both. It was something that influenced my life so profoundly it subconsciously drove me in a direction. Yet when remembered years later it served as a wake-up call allowing me to course correct based on the memory of that experience. It's the chicken or the egg. Which came first is the eternal question, yet both are a reality. In the case of the little girl, was her purpose to prompt me to do something or was her brief life and my part in it what opened me to the idea of healing people? Did it drive me, or did I choose a course based on that event? We will never answer that question; yet it allows us to look at things in our lives from a different perspective.

Rather than labeling events as good or bad we should rather question what impact each will make in our lives. We hold the power to determine how events will shape us, to be who we're supposed to be in life. When I think of my experience's in Catholic school, I realize I never looked at any of it as positive or negative; they were just things that happened. I believe that's probably what saved me. If I had seen peeing my pants in class as a total negative and a failure, that might have caused me to be scared my whole life. If the girl dying had been so traumatic to me that I feared emotional attachment it would have been a negative. Instead, I developed an ability to choose my response to every situation.

I have always had a passion for talking to people, getting out, and doing things. That school experience was obviously interesting with respect to the fact that it was a very controlled and strict environment. I gained a great education, and it pushed me in areas I wasn't comfortable with. As a first grader (today), you never would have been treated that way. Did that environment push me to become the best I could be or was it simply my time to be pushed to be who I could be? It's about choices and questioning those choices. I will explore that more in my book. Anything that happens to you can be an experience— good or bad, it doesn't matter. It's just an experience. What we do with that experience is what defines us.

In this journey we have choices to turn left or right.

Thanksgiving Day 1985 found me on my knees in a 100-year-old log shed digging through two feet of snow to find something to build a fire that might keep me alive through the night. I was living my dream of hunting elk in Idaho, and **it was going to kill me!** My ego had driven me all day to walk through three feet of snow in 14-degree weather. I should've been home with my family having Thanksgiving dinner. My friend the deputy sheriff said, "You can't get lost here," slapped me on the back, sending me off in the wrong direction. This "easy" two-hour walk found me half-frozen, and I lay down in the snow as close to giving up as I'd ever been.

Unable to fire my rifle because it was frozen, I drove my gun into the snow and got up. Thoughts of my son David, born just six months earlier, was all that kept me going. I looked around and decided, "I'm going to go left." Turning left I couldn't see anything except driving snow, it was a total whiteout, at 3:30 in the afternoon. Yet turning to the right everything was clear, I could see fine. It felt like God put His hand in front of my eyes and said, "You're not going that way." Going left would have led back to my vehicle, but something appeared to be telling me that I wasn't going to make it if I went that way.

Now on my knees tending several small fires I had managed to start in the rotted logs of this old cabin, I was worried that I would go to sleep and not wake up, so I set my Casio watch to ring every 20 minutes to keep me from going to sleep. I was scared that I would never wake up, fearing hypothermia would set in. I think it was more carbon monoxide poisoning because I remember being warm at the time. I could see lights in the distance but couldn't hear anything despite being 100 yards from the road.

Forty people were out searching for me and the sheriff had warned the party, "If we don't find him soon, he will be dead." Gary, a friend of mine, joined the search around 8:00 p.m. "Look, there's a flicker of light!" The person riding with him insisted, "That's nothing, just snowmobile lights." Gary stopped to check it out anyway, "Dennis!" he yelled. I fired my last shot stating, "I AM HERE." I would've died 100 yards from the road.

We have choices how we connect to people!

Twenty years ago, I watched a friend of mine dying of prostate cancer. I did not have the guts to go by and see him when I should have as he went through the process. I'm not sure why other than it simply scared me, and I felt helpless. It was a poor choice on my part. Having to live with that decision made me change the way I make those decisions in the future. Dealing with decisions honestly can be one of the biggest miracles.

It hits closest to you when you have one of your best friends faced with mortality. I had coffee with Doug every morning for the last 15 years. He was an alcoholic for 30 years or more. He had not had a drink in nearly 20 years. He did love his coffee, cookies, and cigarettes. I would go by his house in the morning and spend 10 or 15 minutes having a cup of coffee. He told me two years ago that the throat cancer he been treated for three years earlier had come back. The recommended treatment would include cutting out half of his tongue and part of his throat. They gave him six months to live even with that treatment. Doug refused, saying that he did not want to lay in bed having people look over him, and he refused to tell almost everyone else. We discussed a treatment program we put him on a regimen of alternative care. We took him off his cookies and his cigarettes, and he started improving.

In August 2018, Doug's daughter came over from Europe and spent a week with him. He had not even wanted to tell her about the cancer. He confided in me that he would not live to 71. He was 70. Being able to have a great visit with his daughter, Doug started back with his cigarettes and cookies. He had lived a full life and was happy with what he was doing. In October 2018, I was teaching in Santa Fe. Before we left, over coffee he told me that his legs were starting to swell. I told them it was his kidney or heart and we would take a look at it on Monday when I returned.

I had a dream on Friday night that Doug was lying on his back with his right knee bent up. I was comforting him as he died. We returned on Monday from Santa Fe. He normally opened the gate to our house when we returned from a trip. The gate was closed, and Doug was not at home. The family has a cabin about an hour away up the river. On Friday morning my wife and I took a trip to his cabin. They have an old cabin on a beautiful place on the Clearwater River. We walked inside and found an ashtray with one cigarette burned-out to the filter and a small load of wood in a wheelbarrow. Doug was peacefully laying on his back with his right leg bent knee up—the same position I saw him in, in my dream. I walked up and put my hand on his knee and was thankful I had been with him when he died.

Learning to connect the dots of what makes magical things happen.

The miracle of the stories is the evolution of how and why I am at this place in life. It has helped me become connected with who I am becoming, and I am thankful for the energy of the Universe connecting us in an incredibly special way. The goal is to be honest with people and ourselves. The door then is wide open for all possibilities. Truly being connected to your purpose allows you to see miracles every day.

About the Author

Dr. Dennis Harper, DC

Dennis has had a single-minded drive to "change the world" since he was a young boy growing up in Crescent City, California. Coupled with a passion for hunting, fishing and the great outdoors, these things were the driving force behind his decision to attend Chiropractic College and move to Idaho shortly after graduation in 1980. Settling in Orofino, Idaho, he has run a successful practice since 1984.

His desire to genuinely want the best for everyone lead him to serve on the Idaho Chiropractic Board both as a member and president for 12 years. It also kept him constantly looking for better treatment options for his patients. This quest led to the creation of the Harper Restoration Systems, a training company for practitioners interested in innovative, leading edge regenerative treatments using Ozone and Biologic Allograft. This combination of things has given him an uncanny ability to listen to what a patient's body is saying, rather than focusing on what the patient wants to tell him. Dr. Harper says that being in front of a room full of doctors and having just minutes to diagnose and treat some very tough patients really hones your diagnostic skills!

Never one to be stationary and being committed to making a difference continues to drive him to create more and better systems to change the world.

Contact Information:

Email: drharperoz1@gmail.com
Website: www.harperozone.com

LIFE IS A MIRACLE

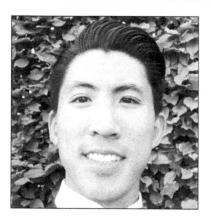

Dr. James Huang

I just turned 40, last year, and that in itself is a miracle from day one.

My parents immigrated to the United States from Taiwan in the late '70s. They came as architecture students with hopes of earning a good education to fulfill the American Dream. My mother was pregnant with her second child in 1979. This became a problem because my older brother was extremely hyperactive. Today, he might have been diagnosed with ADHD and put on medication. As a young baby, my older brother would open up all the cabinets in the house and dump all the contents on the floor. My parents would often find him missing outside across the street in our neighbor's yard. Both my parents were working, and with the stress of finances, their current housing situation, and my brother's ADHD behavior, my mother was planning to terminate the pregnancy. Thankfully, by the grace of God, my mom shared her stress with their church, and the pastor's wife convinced my mother to keep the baby, and I was born on November 2, 1979.

"Everyone deserves to live with a higher quality of life."

Nineteen years later, I became very depressed and physically the weakest I've ever been in my life. I had always been very active growing up and had never had any severe injuries other than just a few scrapes and bruises. But during the winter of 1999, I suffered a severe snowboarding injury that dislocated my shoulder, hip, severely sprained my wrist, and gave me peripheral neuropathy. My medical doctor told me I just had to rest and let it heal on its own. I was also given some muscle relaxers and NSAIDS, received a cortisone shot, and did three months of physical therapy, which helped with the pain, but I had no improvement with the neuropathy or regaining strength.

Six months later, I was still very weak, and my muscles atrophied. I was also given a splint to wear over my sprained wrist and told to wear it every waking minute. I became very weak to the point that I could not even lift a pencil. Eventually, I went into a deep depression. I thought to myself, *I guess this is just how life is going to be. I'm just going to have to live with the neuropathy and weakness in my left arm.* I was about to give up on my recovery when a leader at my church noticed my splint and confidently told me he could help me. He happened to be a sports chiropractor. I was ready to try anything, so I made an appointment and was seen later that week. I didn't know anything about chiropractic care, so I went into the appointment with no expectations. He simply explained that I had compressed joints from my injury, which could lead to neuropathy and decreased function of both my central and peripheral nervous system.

He told me that if he is able to restore normal positioning of my bones, then I would be fine. He had me lay down on this table facedown, and he put his hands on my back, telling me to breathe in and out. As I exhaled, he thrust his hands into my spine. I heard a very loud crack and felt movement in my spine. Soon after, I felt a rush of blood and energy flow through my entire body. He continued to adjust a few more joints, including my shoulder and wrist, and even my hips. I had no idea what he was doing, but it felt great. After he was done treating me, he told me to stop using the wrist splint because I needed to start activating my wrist muscles. He taught me a few wrist extensor exercises.

I couldn't believe it, but I could feel my arm again and I gained my strength back. It was a miracle! I went back for a follow-up appointment two days later, and I was 100% cured. I continued to have regular chiropractic care about every two weeks for maintenance and made a decision to take care of my overall health. I stopped eating fast food, began learning about health and fitness, and started weight training. My depression was gone, and I had never felt better in my life.

"When the impossible becomes possible, we see miracles."

Ten years later, I became a Doctor of Chiropractic (DC), and I see miracles daily in my practice. I believe miracles are when the impossible becomes possible. It wasn't always that way. Early in my practice, I had many difficult patients that I was unable to help. I vividly recall one patient who was having unknown debilitating pain down her leg. She was my last patient of the day, and as I was finishing up my examination, she started having a mild seizure on the table! I was freaking out. I was thinking, *what do I do?!* I remembered from school that seizures are usually caused by an electrical imbalance in the brain, so I ended up grabbing a transcutaneous electrical nerve stimulation (TENS) unit and placed it near the back of her neck. To my surprise, the seizure stopped immediately. Since that moment, two things happened: I decided to devote my life to learning everything I could about the body, and I realized the body is electric!

Fascination with Learning

For the next couple of years, I spent countless hours learning everything I could about the body. I read books on nutrition, quantum physics, and energetic healing. I attended at least 2,000 hours of continuing education to learn how to address sports injuries, neurology, and functional medicine. I fell in love with the concept of healing and became almost addicted to healing not only my own body, but those of my patients. By 2015, I had quickly built a reputation of being the doctor that could help most people with most conditions in my community. Patients would fly in or drive past state lines to see me. This year, I decided to create my own approach and call it the Energy Specific Technique.

The Body is Like a Car

I tell all my patients that the body is like a car. That means that, like a car, there are physical parts that make the body: the muscles, ligaments, joints, tissue, fascia, and bone. A car also has to have fluids: brake and transmission fluid, and oil in the engine. Without the right chemistry, the car won't work. For the body, this is the macronutrients: fats, carbs, and protein, and micronutrients: vitamins and minerals. Lastly, the car has a computer system; that is the brain in the human body, which controls all your muscles and organs and also your ability to taste, see, hear, and smell. In addition to autonomic function, the brain also helps you with balance and coordination and how you control your emotions. So just like a car, if there is no oil in the engine, the car won't run properly. That is the same with the human body. When the body is fully balanced physically, chemically, and mentally, it will function at 100% and healing can occur, and disease will cease to exist. My patients always love to hear this analogy because it makes sense, but they always wonder how. "How are you going to balance out my WHOLE body? How?"

The Body is Electric

As I mentioned earlier, I created my own technique known as the Energy Specific Technique. I've realized that everything is energy, which can be quantified through electricity. After reading *The Body Electric* by Robert O. Becker, I learned that the body is electric and is positively and negatively charged. This means there is a polarity to the body just like the Earth. With this knowledge, you can test the body's electrical field, also known as a biofield or the morphogenic field. From the work of Dr. Springbob, I learned the biofield is an expression of health; the larger the field; the better expression of health. I've found in practice that this field can be anywhere from one inch to eight feet away from the body. In each visit, my main goal is to increase the energetic field as much as possible. This can be done through specific balancing of the body physically, chemically, and mentally.

I'm sure you're wondering what miracle stories I've seen in the clinic using my technique and what that actually looks like clinically. I have had a wide variety of miracle stories over the last 10 years and I'll share seven of them with you.

CASE I: CANCER PATIENT

An 80-year-old female patient presented with thyroid cancer and a tumor around the carotid artery on the right side of her neck since 2018. Symptoms included chronic sinus pain, fatigue, gas, bloating, and diarrhea. Findings revealed weakness of the muscles on the right side. Through muscle testing, we found a sympathetic response over the spleen, thymus, and upper teeth. Her biofield measured about 11 inches from her body. Through the Energy Specific Technique, I determined that she was having a poor flow of electricity around her mouth due to her upper metal dentures. I referred her to a holistic dentist in Berkeley—Dr. Hites, and he replaced the metal dentures with non-metal ones. After getting treated once a month for five months, she reported her tumor had reduced 75%, and all of her original symptoms have gone away.

CASE II: FROZEN SHOULDER

A 55-year-old male presented to the clinic with frozen shoulder on the left side with no history of trauma. The patient recalled waking up with the inability to move the shoulder more than 90 degrees and pain with abduction at a 9/10. Through muscle testing and the Energy Specific Technique, it was determined the patient was sensitive to wireless radiation. After about a month of treatment with this protocol, I was able to restore the shoulder to full range of motion and the patient was pain-free.

CASE III: PHANTOM PAIN

A 30-year-old female nurse presented to the office with

phantom pain down her left leg with moderate pain of 8/10. She was unable to walk or sleep without pain. She was seen by orthopedists, MDs, and had X-rays, blood tests, and MRIs. All tests resulted in normal findings. She even was treated by multiple chiropractors. One main finding during diagnosis was the inability for her to fire multiple muscles at a time and activate her default mode network. After one treatment, 80% of her symptoms were resolved and after the second visit, she was 100% better.

CASE IV: ALCOHOL ALLERGY

A 37-year-old male suffered for five years from an allergic reaction to alcohol, which would cause a skin rash all over his body. He had seen many medical specialists and all labs tested normal. I found there was an emotional component related to the allergic reaction. Through the energy specific protocols, we were able to reset the limbic system and bring his body back to a parasympathetic state. The patient later stated that he drank some alcohol at a bachelor party and had no response to it and was completely symptom-free.

CASE V: NEVERENDING HEADACHES

A 9-year-old female suffered for two years with chronic headaches, projectile vomiting, and severe sensitivity to barley. She would get headaches 6 to 7 days a week that would last for 4 to 5 hours a day. The patient presented with extreme muscle weakness in all her limbs and was exacerbated when near any Bluetooth activated device. After a year of treatment she has had zero headaches and is no longer allergic to barley. In addition, all her limbs are functional, and all muscle weakness has subsided. Her well-being is no longer exacerbated by Bluetooth technology.

CASE VI: FLU SYMPTOMS, ALLERGIES, AND DIFFICULTY BREATHING

A 40-year-old female presented with flu-like symptoms: fever, fatigue, sore throat, dry cough, nausea, headaches, and difficulty breathing for two months with no improvement. She also presented with itchy eyes and a runny nose, which she claimed was from seasonal allergies that she dealt with for years. After two visits all flu-like symptoms were resolved, but allergy symptoms still remained. After five weeks of treatments all of her symptoms resolved, and she is able to enjoy the outdoors without any issues.

CASE VII: SNORING, SLEEP APNEA, AND JAW PAIN

A 30-year-old male musician presented with headaches, high blood pressure, anxiety, anemia, extreme jaw pain, sleep apnea, and snoring. History of trauma to the jaw from a car accident made it very difficult for the patient to breathe through his nose. This patient also was known to snore and have sleep apnea for three years. He had seen many TMJ specialists with no results and had constant pain of 8/10 in his jaw and 5/10 in his neck. I used a combination of the Nasal Specific Technique and the Energy Specific Technique to restore function back to this patient. After only six treatments over the course of three months this patient has fully recovered from all of his symptoms, and his pain levels went down to a 1/10 for both the jaw and the neck.

What I've learned over the last ten years is this:

Miracles don't have to be difficult, just possible.

About the Author

Dr. James Huang

James has trained in many chiropractic techniques (Zone Technique, Applied Kinesiology, Neuro Emotional Technique, Cranial Facial Release, SOT, and other modalities). As a young practitioner, he found it very difficult to apply all these techniques on a patient during a visit. So after years of practice, he has come up with his own protocol system, the Energy Specific Technique, that has been able to address the whole body in a very fast and effective way. He gets between 50%–70% improvement of the patient's symptoms after the first visit. His protocols have been very effective in treating patients with vertigo, concussions, headaches, sciatica, herniated discs, frozen shoulder, carpal tunnel, and even the common flu. He specializes in relieving headaches, migraines, TMJ, sciatica, sports injuries, carpal tunnel, and nerve pain.

Contact Information:

Holistic Chiropractic and Kinesiology
Website: www.drjameshuang.com
Facebook: holisticsportscare
Instagram: @drjameshuang
Email: drjameshuangdc@gmail.com

THE ANGEL OF DEATH

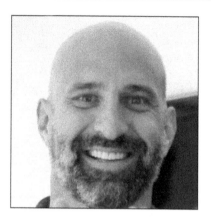

Brad Axelrad

As my mother spoke, I knew immediately that something was wrong. Normally upbeat and confident, she spoke with bewildered hesitation as she told me my father had some trouble finding his way home. My heart dropped into my stomach. My father, the man whom I have always looked up to for strength, does not get lost in the small community he knows so well. You'd find him at the gym at 4:00 and 5:00 every morning. He was a pretty healthy dude and took good care of himself.

We both agreed that she had to get him to the doctor right away to see what was wrong. After a few days of tests, we found out he had a golf ball-sized tumor in his brain. It was malignant and had to be surgically removed immediately. After the surgery came chemotherapy and radiation. My father was given one year to live. He slipped away in four short months and I watched my father take his last breath on October 19th, 2005.

As I held my father's hand in the ICU, I watched his spirit lift from his body. It truly was the most difficult, yet amazing experience to see his transition into the spiritual realm. I am grateful to have been at his side during those last moments. To see my father at peace helped me find the strength to cope with my loss and make a transition into a deeper, more spiritual life.

Less than two days later, I found myself again in the most loving place I have ever experienced, The Hoffman Institute in St. Helena, California. Seven months earlier I had enrolled in their three-day workshop. The timing was magical, as I needed a place to grieve and reconnect with my spiritual self. After I completed the healing workshop, I drove two hours south to the Bay Area for my father's life celebration. I was petrified to face the reality that my father was no longer with us. Once I arrived, that all changed as it became a joyous celebration of life as I witnessed how much this man had impacted others.

After a few days of decompression, I drove home to Orange County down the lonesome Highway 5. I realized it was up to me to leave a legacy as my father did. As my awareness of this purpose opened up, I simultaneously went into the darkest months of my life. I had never felt so alone, so scared, and so raw. I was regularly overcome with sudden outbursts of crying. I missed my father very much.

During my dark days and nights, alone and hibernating, I could feel the heavy burden and guilt from many years of not being around my father. The shame. The regret. The despair. I ran from my family and myself to Orange County from the San Francisco Bay Area. Geographic healing was something I knew well; I was an expert at it. As angry and resentful as I was at my father for not being perfect, I had never missed him more. Even with people around me, supporting me, loving me, I still felt very alone. Emotional pain was now part of my everyday life. As tears rolled down my face and as I was beaten into submission, begging the Universe for relief, I realized I had nothing left and had no choice but to surrender.

Mortality—my father's and my own—woke me up. It made me suddenly conscious of how precious every moment is.

With the nudge from my father, I started my first business at 10 years old. He always inspired me to go after my dreams and desires. Midweek powder days in the Tahoe Mountains 50 days a winter was the norm. Racing motocross was my passion.

Ultimately, I became a championship-winning semi-professional motocross racer, traveling the West Coast, following my passion, and making money.

Starting my first real business at 19, then selling another by 26, I took the risks and faced my fear, always saying yes to my dream. However, his passing shook me to my bones and rocked me to my core. All of the self-indulgence became meaningless. I knew something HAD to change. As I was literally beaten down to my knees, begging the Universe for some salvation, crying and wailing in my hallway, I pleaded, "Please show me my purpose! I cannot die like my dad did with his voice still in him!"

My purpose showed up when I realized I had nothing left but to use my body as a vessel of service to humanity. My entire life of self-indulgence had left me feeling empty. Only this time, it was a mirror held up to my face. In that moment of self-realization, I finally realized my powerful abilities of manifestation. I am a natural-born leader, just as my father was, and I had to use my knowledge and passion to create a better life for myself and others around me. I immediately embraced this role and sought out a way to be of service.

Now my Dad was a uniquely powerful man, but he never really stepped into his purpose or dharma. He seemed sort of stuck in limbo, never fully in his power. We could all feel a sort of quiet desperation, and I was committed to not living a life without miracles.

To initiate my higher purpose and to give back to humanity, I decided to host monthly Hoffman Institute graduate gatherings in my home. I met many powerful, positive people through Hoffman, and I wanted to continue the energy. By leading these meetings for two years, I was inspired to host a study group on quantum physics. I had been studying this material for the last few years, and it resonated with my core beliefs and being. By embracing and applying this deep, truth-filled material, I realized that my desires were obtainable.

Two weeks later, I hosted our first study group where I led a small group through an evening of connection and processes. By the second week, people were driving from a hundred miles away to attend the meetings! Within four weeks, we doubled in size. Within eight weeks, 40 of us were visited by NBC Nightly News, and my entire life changed! USC News later did a piece on us as well as a local PBS affiliate television station, CBC News Canada, the Orange County Register and the Los Angeles Times.

After having produced over 150 live events with some of the biggest thought and business leaders on the planet, I was aligned with something much more meaningful and contributory. Self-indulgence was a thing of the past; transforming the lives of the thousands who attended and the next courageous souls who said YES to themselves was my future.

And to top it all off, I was invited in 2010 to meet twice a year with other transformational leaders as a Founding Member of ATL SoCal (Association of Transformational Leaders), a forum for individuals of significant influence in artistic, academic, social, political, corporate and humanitarian endeavors, devoted to doing transformational work in their respective fields.

Life was good! But it can change in an instant.

Taking a prescribed medication in 2011, I nearly died. Like so many of us, I was quick to take medication instead of getting to the root cause of the problem and choosing a more holistic approach. With my liver swelling huge in my ribcage, literally rubbing against the inside of it, I was certain I destroyed my liver. I faced mortality once again—this time, my own. I could barely eat anything that was fatty for months without it irritating it. It took many years for my liver to heal.

Had I known that there were other ways to heal the root problem, leaky gut that was creating the Candida, I would have tried another way. I took a very strong anti-fungal to get rid of the white spots on my skin. Ever seen those? It's a fungus. This could have been easily fixed with diet and a few other changes. My gut flora was compromised from all the ibuprofen I took while racing motocross. It helped me deal with the constant pain I had inflicted on myself with motocross and extreme sports all those years. Poor food choices and the American diet didn't help much either.

Now I've had many injuries, health scares and surgeries in my life, but this was hands down the scariest. As I researched liver transplants, reality set in. If I did indeed need one, I was very far down the list and highly unlikely to receive a new liver. This prompted me to rethink many things in my life, really getting me to face the biggest dragon of my life—my own mortality.

Twenty-four months of sober celibacy deep in the Colorado mountains helped me gain incredible clarity. I spent many hours in solitude, asking God and the Universe to show me a message. Many days in deep contemplation… Many hours of conversations with mentors, coaches, and consultants… Many deep dives with numerous shamans, finding a deeper level of connection to my own divinity and others…

Fast forward several years, I've been heavily focused on gut healing detoxing, doing many cleanses, liver, gallbladder, candida, and am feeling much better. Integrating the best of technology, nutrition, supplementation, regenerative medicine, and anything else that will help me heal. I will not make the same mistake my father did, thinking he was doing the right things for his health. He did his best with the knowledge he had at the time; I will know for sure and apply what is proven to work, not what I think works.

As my purpose continues to unfold and Steven E and I build out Wake Up Worldwide Events (centers around the world of monthly gatherings focused on biohacking, anti-aging and longevity), I expand with love of purpose and humanity. And the cool thing is, I'm exposed to all the latest and greatest modalities for optimal living.

I feel my whole self being guided and living connected to the universal energy. Facing death can do that to a person.

There is a knowingness now that we are ever-expanding beings with infinite creating potential. I am tapped into the flow and am using it to benefit others locally and globally. As our membership base grows, we are spreading our message around the world. My life is flourishing and expanding. I am joyous, healthy and experience bliss on a regular basis. People around me are feeling and experiencing it, too. I have become a servant of the flow!

Don Miguel Ruiz, the author of the blockbuster bestselling book *The Four Agreements*, was my first guest on my Face Your Dragon Podcast. He so brilliantly states the angel of death can really serve us to open and reminds us to live in the present moment, as it's the only moment we have; our time here really is short and can be taken away in an instant.

And as I like to say to my clients and podcast listeners at Face Your Dragon, "What you are most resisting and most afraid of are the very things that will set you free. It's your money-maker, your gift to humanity, and your purpose on the planet." Lean in and allow the angel of death to be your motivation. Leverage your fear into your great work in the world and say yes to your highest calling. The world is waiting!

As I surrender to being an instrument of the Universe, I watch my life and legacy unfold, standing in my fear and using it for good. I am forever grateful for the pain of my father's passing and the wonderful character he instilled in me. I allow him to guide me on a regular basis and watch my dreams manifest. I am honored to be on the leading edge of this movement as humanity wakes up to this new paradigm.

My purpose in life is to create transformation in communities and in leaders worldwide, helping them to live from their deepest heart, as healthy as possible.

I am beyond thankful for another chance at life and to be healthy and happy.

As my impact grows and expands, so does my humility and gratitude.

About the Author

Brad Axelrad

Brad's produced over 150 live events with top business leaders and best-selling authors. His Face Your Dragon brand consults visionary entrepreneurs. Co-Founder of the Wake Up Worldwide Events, centers around the world of monthly gatherings focused on biohacking, anti-aging, and longevity.

Founding member of the Association of Transformational Leaders SoCal, seen on national media outlets. On his Face Your Dragon Podcast he interviews icons including don Miguel Ruiz, Arielle Ford, and JP Sears.

Contact Information:

Brad Axelrad
brad@faceyourdragon.com
714.330.4031
faceyourdragon.com

THE ULTIMATE SOFTWARE FOR THE BODY

Natural Energy Medicine for the Body, Mind & Spirit

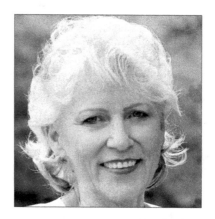

Debbie Orr

True health can be achieved when we can identify and balance distortions in the energy field of the body. I have worked in the field of energy medicine for over 30 years and it has been nothing short of a miracle to see lives changed when the distortions (or corrupted programming) of the biofield of the body are restored and balanced allowing the body to function as our creator designed it to. Remember, the human body is not one device but two. The physical body is a very sophisticated bio-electrical-mechanical and completely autonomous machine. It will wear out, break, and just quit someday. Then you have the person, the living component that lives in this machine as long as it continues to function. Our traditional healthcare professionals address the machine not the person. We are able to fix the person only when we can fix the machine. In reality, the physical body is a very sophisticated autonomous machine that requires little to no outside help unless it becomes corrupted or damaged.

The human body is made up of trillions of cells, and these cells perform countless biochemical functions daily so the body can maintain health. So you may ask what orchestrates all these biochemical functions in the body. It is energy (frequency) that provides the signals. Remember, energy is simply the ability of a physical system to change. Everything gives and receives energy, and that includes every cell in the body. The body is a crystalline substrate and coherent light and energy are critical components for proper function.

We are just starting to recognize, understand, and investigate the profound role light and frequency plays in regulating and maintaining health in the human body. Traditional medicine today basically ignores the importance of the body's energy fields and why people like you and me seek answers on how to restore energy, frequency, and proper signaling in the body. When we utilize natural energy medicine tools, programming can be restored and those energy blocks resolved, then healing is a natural process that is an ongoing function for which we were designed.

You Can Talk to the Body

Just imagine that you can talk to the body. Our cells have their own communication system and they have a memory. Did you know that everything in our world has its own identifiable frequency? We could describe that as having their own unique, energetic thumbprint. For example, oak pollen has its own unique frequency, gluten has its own frequency, Clorox has its own frequency, as does each of your own organs and tissues within your body. Even emotions have their own frequency. Are you familiar with the science of homeopathy? This science is based on frequencies.

The science of acupuncture utilizes the frequency highways of the body called the meridians to help balance and support the body to help it heal. But just as you speak and understand your own native language the body has its own language and it listens and responds when we speak to it with the proper information or in its language. There are different tools used to access and communicate with the frequency information system of the body but **finding the right tools** that speak precisely to the body is paramount for the best outcomes.

To help you better understand; let's look at the computer, which was designed after our own bodies. It uses an information system of data and requires a main CPU to organize that data, so it is accessible by the user. But what happens when the computer gets corrupted and infected with viruses or the hard drive becomes overloaded with bad information? To put it simply, the programming becomes broken and it slows down and does not work efficiently, and if bad enough, the computer just stops working. Fortunately, developers who know the right programming language have designed software to help remove those pesky viruses and malware that have invaded and corrupted the programming of your computer and disrupted the proper information exchange.

An amazing thing happens after you run that repair software. The computer we thought was useless comes back to life and now functions properly. A miracle, right? The same thing happens in our bodies. Simply put, our bodies are an information system. But remember that in healthcare we are not talking about our conscious memory or the person that you know as you, we are talking about the **bio-electrical-mechanical machine** that we call the human body that we live in. We believe that primarily within our central nervous system we contain stored data, called body memory, programming that utilizes that data, and an operating system that manages it all. And we know that this body data and programming can learn, that is how we learn to walk and talk.

Just like all data it can become corrupted, which is why after some forms of trauma, toxins, or pathogens, we can lose that data and have to relearn how to walk and talk or fight a disease or recognize and digest a food properly and so on. The body can become infected with misinformation that cause all sorts of malfunction and inappropriate responses in the body. These malfunctions and inappropriate responses can then cause different symptoms, some minor and others very serious. In essence, the body needs its own form of software or reprogramming to help support, reorganize, and repair its own software. We believe that it is possible that **the root cause of poor health** may be due to the corruption of our body data, programming, and our operating system.

Natural energy medicine is the only healthcare procedure that is specifically designed to address health in this manner. Please understand, this process does not diagnose a disease or attempt to treat medical conditions. But when the body can receive the appropriate information it needs from a number of sources such as living organic foods and nutrients, pure living water, exercise, oxygen, including coherent low-level laser light and other supportive frequencies that all support the body's normal function, then the body on its own acts on that information, and then proper function can be restored. **The body is a miraculous machine** capable of homeostasis. It has its own language and wants and needs precise and proper information it can understand, interpret, and act on to thrive and heal. Balance, balance, balance is the priority.

True natural light and frequency therapy is a very complex and multifaceted healthcare system that is not easily explained or defined as these explanations are hidden in the field of quantum physics, which is still beyond the full understanding of modern science. However, just because we cannot understand how it works does not mean that we cannot understand the way it works and how to use it. You may not know how to build a car, but you can still drive one. Just as traditional Chinese medicine and acupuncture are very old systems of medicine being rediscovered, so is light and frequency therapy.

Heliotherapy (light therapy) was practiced by physicians in ancient cultures in Egypt, Greece, China, and India to address many conditions. In the 1660s, Isaac Newton separated light with a prism and discovered the visible spectrum. In the 1890s, a Danish physician, Dr. Niels Finsen, pioneered light therapy. So successful was his work in treating skin tuberculosis with light that he was awarded the Nobel Prize in 1903. Works of innovators like these and others provide us with sufficient empirical evidence of the value of light and frequency in medicine. The scientific evidence for this rests in quantum physics and the color theory, the photoelectric effect first discovered by Hertz, and the theory of light elucidated by Albert Einstein.

To better understand how light and information is utilized by the body, we want to have a grasp of a few key processes. Biomodulation is defined as changing the natural biochemical response of a cell or tissue within the normal range of its function, stimulating the cell's innate metabolism, thereby allowing the cell to heal itself. Photo biomodulation is the process of biomodulating tissue with a photon or activating or inhibiting cellular function by applying a specific photon that is transferred to a light receptor within the tissues (the biological chromophore). This is a very powerful form of informational medicine and delivers not only an energy stimulus but information as well.

Einstein stated many years prior to the discovery of the LASER (Light Amplification by Stimulated Emission of Radiation) that the internal cell-to-cell communication of the body was performed through coherent light. As science discovered how to manufacture LASER (coherent) light, light therapy went from general health support to specific correctional healthcare procedures. The process of **photobiomodulation (low-level laser therapy)** requires a very specific form of light, (coherent, polarized and collimated) a very specific wavelength (color-635), and a very specific power density (brightness less than 5mw). If all of these properties of light are not exactly correct, the light may have a variety of effects on the body but photobiomodulation is not one of them.

A form of light therapy that is specifically designed to produce photobiomodulation of all tissue would more accurately be described as informational medicine or the foundation component of natural energy medicine. It is considered the foundation because it is the carrier or delivers all other types of informational medicine of which natural energy medicine is composed. Photo biomodulation is valuable in stimulating neuroplastic changes in the brain. BioLight's laser systems utilize true coherent, polarized, and collimated light at less than 5mw of power, making it very safe and effective. This utilizes the

635Hz wavelength, allowing one to activate the light receptors (chromophore) plus the very unique ability to pulse at 120M pulses per second, which makes it one of the most precise low level therapy laser systems available. Both the PTL laser systems and the Qi-5 Body Scan system use high functioning lasers to provide information to the body.

I want to share a few miraculous real life stories of people with significant health challenges who were fortunate enough to experience this form of information, self-correction, and balance within their body that changed their lives. I know you will be touched as I share the hope these people experienced.

Miracle 1

"I finally have my life back," says 13-year-old Alisa, who lived in South Carolina, after going through a series of scans and laser sessions. Her story started when she was just 11 years old and she started experiencing over a matter of months headaches and pain all through her body. Everything she ate except a very few foods affected her very negatively. Alisa would also throw up every day and she was unable to sleep. Her heart would race and pound constantly. She basically had become a shut-in and stayed in her room most of the time, trapped by her own body's dysfunction.

Her mother started searching and taking her from doctor to doctor with test after test, but there were no answers. The mother recanted that her daughter was even fired as a patient by a doctor because they were totally stumped and could not figure out what the issue was for Alisa. Over the next two years, her life became more and more restricted and she basically had a few baby food items she could tolerate that became her very limited food source, if you can even imagine.

In January of 2019, they finally had to take Alisa out of school because she was absent so much and just could not function there. Her mother recounts how her heart was breaking as she watched her daughter become a shadow of the person she once was, and even worse that they had no hope of bringing their daughter back to health and vitality again. They were in a hopeless state.

Then miraculously, they found a BioLight practitioner.

As Alisa walked in, the practitioner observed that she was withdrawn, frail, and pretty much despondent. The practitioner used the Qi-5 Balance and the PTL II Low Level Light Therapy laser system to help identify distortions in her information system and support the body's energy field. At the end of the session, Alisa had perked up and she turned to her mother and said, "Mom, my heart is not pounding anymore." That was a first sign of many changes to come. That night, Alisa slept through the night and her pain was significantly reduced. She also reported the nonstop headache was gone. Their hope soared at this point. After that, Alisa and her mom continued to work with the practitioner. The next miracle was that she was able to attend in just a few short weeks a soccer camp she was longing to attend but had little hope before. By the fall, she was able to return to school.

This young lady has totally blossomed, and her body has begun on its own the journey back to balance and health. We have to remember the body is the real healing tool. When we can help support the bioenergetic body by identifying energetic distortions and imbalances and support it with good information, the body is able to take over and miraculously bring itself back online. The body innately knows how to heal when it has the right information. The body is wonderfully and miraculously made.

Miracle 2

Diana was a young woman in her 20s with Down syndrome who had been damaged in a surgery gone wrong for an inner ear issue. She was a talented dancer and had even been featured on a local TV station for her talent in spite of her disability. But when she started having balance issues, it was recommended that she have a surgery to correct it. Sadly, when she came out of surgery and while in recovery, she started having grand mal seizures and could not even drink or eat anything without it triggering a seizure. They ran all sorts of test and could not figure out what went wrong. Her parents took her from doctor to doctor trying to find answers for their precious daughter. It had become critical and a neurologist who was in the same office with a doctor who used the BioLight system recommended the family to him as a last resort, knowing of other cases in which he had seen miraculous results.

The neurologist expressed to him that he did not feel she would make it through the next 48 hours without a miracle and asked him if he would see Diana on Christmas Eve day. He saw her that very day and started her with some basic balancing visits with the laser and her body calmed down. She stabilized and could drink water without triggering a seizure and she was able to sleep. The doctor recommended they return the next day because he knew she could not wait until after the holidays. Diana returned daily for the next five days. Each day she responded positively as her body began to balance out and calm down. Her seizures grew more and more seldom, and she was able to start slowly eating again. She continued to have other issues such as vibrations in her eyes and would have little quivering events, but every week she would improve more and more. It was truly a miracle this young woman is still with us, but she is thriving three years later and is back to her dancing with so much joy in her heart. Her parents know that the doctor and the PTL laser were their answer to much prayer and they had received a miracle that changed all their lives forever.

BioLight Technologies specialize in bioenergetic biofield assessment technology, low-level laser technology, and complementary products to support the energetic body in its journey to balance and wellness. It is exciting to be able to unlock and stimulate the innate healing ability of the human body utilizing these innovative systems and products. BioLight's expertise is in the scientific integration of complementary alternative medicine and holistic wellness philosophies such as acupuncture, chiropractic care, homeopathy, naturopathy, applied kinesiology, message, nutrition, and laser therapy. We bring together the best of traditional Eastern health philosophies, modern technology, and related mind/body science, providing a safe, non-invasive, and natural approach for optimizing health and promoting wellness. BioLight systems do not diagnose or treat medical conditions.

About the Author

Debbie Orr

Debbie is the CEO of BioLight Technologies. She has worked in natural energy medicine for 25 years. She has extensive education and training in natural energy medicine and has trained hundreds of doctors and holistic medicine practitioners. BioLight Technologies manufactures and distributes the Qi-5 Balance system (eight-channel scan and laser) and the PTL low-level laser therapy systems, along with a complete line of bioenergetic products. BioLight utilizes a truly integrative approach incorporating the next generation of lasers and frequency information systems that go far beyond others systems on the market. BioLight's integrative systems will change how you address whole body wellness as we stand firmly in the center of true energy medicine. We are proud to introduce the next generation of natural energy medicine for the future of humanity.

Contact Information:

Debbie Orr, CEO
BioLight Technologies
www.biolighttechnologies.com
debbie@biolighttechnologies.com
877-229-3000

AYAHUASCA, A HEALING TRIP IN THE JUNGLE

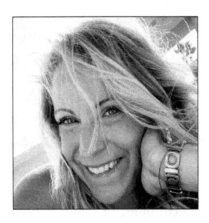

Lisa Marie Crawford

Living in the west, we have become accustomed to leaning on Western medical practices that may include doctors, pharmaceuticals, and surgeries. Often times the things that are prescribed to us are based on Western philosophies, many of which tend to treat the symptoms we are experiencing rather than the core root of what is actually going on in our body, heart, or mind. This can lead to countless doctor visits, multiple medications being prescribed that we may not even need nor should be taking to begin with, and potentially unnecessary surgeries. Just because this is the way that institutions train doctors does not mean that they are the only way or the right way to approach our individual care. We are literally being marketed to around every corner all the time for things that aren't necessarily there to serve us.

Personally, I found that by actively seeking and participating in alternative medicinal and holistic approaches to my overall health, I was better able to truly resolve the challenge I faced on a core level as opposed to continuing on with prescriptions and doing what was presented to me at the time as an inevitable spine surgery. I used many unconventional holistic modalities in my journey of healing but will focus on Ayahuasca here for the purpose of this book.

I was 27 years old at the time, physically active with zero back issues and no physical accidents to date. Yet one day in September of 2007, I found myself stuck and hinged sideways at the hip, immobilized with my back muscles tightened and contorted while experiencing the worst pain I have ever endured in my life. I had no idea what was wrong, and I was terrified. I went to a chiropractor who issued an MRI that gave me the results of what had happened. I was diagnosed with three herniated discs at L3, L4, and L5, bulging in varying degrees of large millimeter proportions, bad disc degeneration, severe spinal stenosis, pinched nerves, and arthritis all over my lower lumbar. The analysis was super scary as I had never experienced anything like this before. The chiropractor said that he could treat it and I accepted his services without any further review of my current situation from any other specialists at the time.

Finally after a month of torture I seemed to be free from my physical prison. My back muscles had relaxed, I was no longer stuck in a sideways position, and the pain had subsided. I thought I was good to go and chalked this incident up to a one-time occurrence and resumed my life as normal pre-injury. Unfortunately, this turned out to be the first serious incident of many that occurred over a 10-year period, which were as painful and disabling, or even more so, as the first incident. From 2007 to 2016 my back went out four to six times per year, resulting in all of the same trauma, pain, and symptoms I had experienced the first time including strained walking, sitting and sleeping. The episodes usually lasted six days to two weeks. I thought this was nothing compared to the first time and just tolerated it. It had become my new norm. I never let the episodes completely take me down and I just kept muddling through them. I was in pain and misery during the outages and felt great, completely normal, active and comfortable the rest of the time as if nothing was wrong. That first year or so I just went back to my chiropractor for treatment until each outage was under control.

Eventually I went to my family care doctor for a review of my situation. He said past having a spine surgery and/or just managing the outages there wasn't much I could do. He gave me painkillers and muscle relaxers to help mitigate the pain and make me a bit more comfortable with each incident.

During an episode a few years later, a friend suggested a pain management clinic that he had been going to for treatment of his back. What they wanted to do seemed completely counterintuitive to me. They wanted to burn my nerve endings like an ablation so that I wouldn't feel any pain. I'm sorry, what?! Isn't that how I am supposed to know that something is wrong, my nerves sending a signal to my brain? No thanks! Then they wanted to do cortisone injections into my spine of which you're only supposed to have like three in your lifetime I hear. Hard pass! Then they too prescribed pain medication and muscle relaxants. All of these things were just temporary band-aids that addressed my symptoms not my core cause. I denied all of the treatments except the pain medication.

This would prove detrimental for me later as I started to take the pain medication recreationally and then got hooked on them for a period of time. Now not only was I suffering through back outages every other month or so, but I was now having to deal with all of the side effects from the pain medication mentally, physically, emotionally, and spiritually. I felt trapped.

I knew I had to do something and fast! Years prior, I had heard of people doing Ayahuasca plant medicine ceremonies in Peru as a healing modality. I decided to embark upon this journey of plant-based healing. I had never injured my spine that I was aware of, so I figured it had to be a physical manifestation of something else that was going on. I wasn't sure what this could be as I had a very successful career, great loving family and friends, and had created a good life for myself.

In May 2017, I set off to Peru in search of the holistic healing plant medicine. Ayahuasca is one of the most potent psychedelics known to man that is all-natural from the Earth. Tribes in this region have been using it as a mind, body, and spirit healer for centuries. After flying into Iquitos, I took a bus ride and multiple boats to journey up the Amazon River to a remote village that has been doing Ayahuasca ceremonies for Westerners since the 1980s. The village is deep in the jungle, literally in the middle of nowhere; no electricity, cell or Wi-Fi services, no running water and thus, we bathed in the river. We slept on boards under nets in little huts, and were surrounded by some of the biggest mosquitos, cockroaches, deadly spiders, and lethal snakes to have ever inhabited the planet. I wondered what the hell I had gotten myself into. The journalist, Peter Gorman, lived and studied for decades with the village family that was hosting me. He would come to be a part of my story in the coming years.

I did five Ayahuasca ceremonies in the two weeks I was there. Every ceremony was completely different than the next. Some ceremonies were fun and enlightening and others scary, yet still packed full of love, light, and lessons. Mother Ayahuasca is a healing medicine, not a drug, connecting you to yourself, mother earth, the Universe, God, and all sapient beings. She shows you everything you want to see, everything you don't want to see, and everything you didn't know you needed to see. She brings your subconscious to your conscious. It's like doing 20 years of therapy within each four- to eight-hour session, safely guided by a shaman in a traditional setting and ceremony in the depths of the very alive jungle.

We went down the Amazon collecting the ingredients and helped the shaman make our elixir so that each of our essence, individual intentions and love, are in the batch. The ceremonies began at 8:00 p.m. and went until midnight. After you drink a nasty tasting cup of the plant cocktail, you lay back on your mat and for the next eight hours are immersed in a blockbuster movie like visual feast of your life and everything that has occurred to date. You get to see, explore, and experience all that is great and all that has been ailing you and why. She provides evidence and answers to all of the questions you seek, some without knowing you were seeking them.

The medicine is so gentle, yet so brutally honest. If you fight the medicine and the experience, she will fight back and you will get your ass whooped until you just let go and follow the medicine where it needs to take you, and where you need to go. Your ego has no place here and will eventually be abolished in one of the ceremonies. You have to be willing to step into the pain as well as accept and receive all of the beauty you are shown. You go into a vision for a while and then surface. And then drop back in, continuing to dive deeper and deeper until you see and feel the clarity that the medicine is helping you to discover. She finds the scars and soothes them so you can step beyond your limitations. It's okay to hurt during the process but not to suffer. She will test your boundaries and have you grapple with the issues but never more than you can handle. Just because you may not be getting what you want doesn't mean you're not getting what you need. You learn to trust and work with the medicine and the healing it is trying to do. It takes a lot of courage to sit with and be with this medicine.

In each of my very different Ayahuasca experiences, Mother A and I did a lot of work on my past and my relationship with each version/identity of myself as I lived my seemingly many lives within this life, thus far. I experienced my fears, joys, troubles, losses, wins, pain, happiness, love, and wisdom. We explored the things that I had glommed onto over the years as well as reexperienced things I had deemed true that were given to me by other people (and not myself) along my path to better understand the impacts they were having on me and my life. We scanned and explored my physical, mental, spiritual and emotional health. We looked at habits, patterns, and impulses that were no longer serving me, and why they had originated to begin with, which allowed me to break free from them. Mother A showed me that it's okay to feel or plead guilty about seemingly negative things I had done, but there was no need to feel shame about who I was at different times in my life. I had the pleasure of rediscovering oneness and reintroducing myself to myself, restored to my natural, transparent, and authentic self.

Understandings were made, blocks were broken through, blind spots were brought to light, old energies were cleared, unconditional love for myself, love for others, and love in general were all very present. My heart was burst wide open, my faith restored, forgiveness to myself and others freely given, my soul unchained and untethered, my emotions balanced, clarity gained, and my physical body tensions free, relaxed, and open.

After experiencing, exploring, clearing and healing all of the emotional and spiritual happenings in my world and truly understanding and integrating those things, Mother A then went to work on my spine. The meditative and lucid dreaming state, combined with profound visual effects served as a facilitator in connecting the mind and body to work in harmony with my physical body healing.

I released all of the tension, restrictions, tightness, and guarding that I had been doing trying to guard and protect my back. We worked together on loosening constrictions, relaxing muscles, opening up spaces for energy flow, and redirected breath, oxygen, and blood to assist in healing. We analyzed my chakras and cleared blockages in them so that they could return to their free flowing state. We healed cells in my body that had been damaged. She taught me patience, tolerance and understanding. She helped me create a healing ecosystem in which I could nurture and love my back. She showed me how I spoke to my back, "Why this outage now, this is the worst time ever with all that I have to do. I hate you, back! God, why are you so weak? Stop causing this pain to me." I saw my inner dialogue towards not only my back but other areas as well that were perpetuating issues and gained understanding of the impact of our words and thoughts.

And then we turned my words to, "I love you, back. You are so strong. Thank you for supporting me. What can I give you to help you?" I started to work with my back and not against it. I felt compassion and sympathy. I wanted to do everything I could to help it especially now that I felt I was capable of doing so. I gained the knowledge that our bodies are capable of healing themselves. Experiencing all of this in such a real life like fashion and integrating it on such a cellular level was the ultimate in overall healing.

After returning from the jungle, I had a full year freed of any back outages, free from pain, medication and sleeping pills. I was re-creating a healthier life, giving continuous love and support to my spine. Then boom! Another outage hit. I immediately went and got an MRI to see what had happened and if I had created any real change during my trip to the jungle. The results were significant. The L4 disc that the multiple surgeons told me was F'd and would never heal on its own, had reabsorbed back into my spine, and was no longer herniated/extruded. The L3 disc had partially reabsorbed, and the L5 disc had become slightly worse, which is why my back went out. I was ecstatic! I had healed my really bad disc and partially healed the other. If this was possible with these two, I could certainly do it again and my body could heal L5 as well.

I had such a magical and life changing experience in the jungle that I went back in May of 2019, this time with a documentarian in toe and a handful of close friends. Now, that I knew what the many planet and animal medicines that are in the jungle were capable of, I wanted to go back to share the experience and benefits with my friends and ultimately with you and everyone through my documentary. I was eager to return to the jungle to see my new friends there and to do a checkup of sorts with Mother A and seek care for my remaining L5 disc.

On April 21, 2020, I had a visit with a renowned spine surgeon. As she examined my four MRIs from the last five years, she was looking at them and me with curiosity. She then asked me what I had done between 2015 and 2020. Before I answered, I asked her why she was asking. She proceeded to show me on the imaging how severe my spine had become as of 2015 versus the near perfect spine I had now as of my most recent MRI. "Lisa, this is extraordinary!" she exclaimed. Then went on to say that all three of my discs have completely reabsorbed back into my spine and were no longer herniated/extruded. She also shared that even my severe spinal stenosis had almost completely healed except in one small part of my spine.

She emphasized how remarkable this was especially with the large millimeter proportions of herniations and how severe my spinal stenosis was. She said that if she had met me in 2015, she would have had me into surgery like that day and that now there was zero reason for me to have any sort of spine surgery at all. She went on to say that people don't usually get these kind of results without actually having a major spine surgery, so she asked me again what I had done to heal my back. I shared with her the holistic quest I had been on and all of the modalities

I incorporated. She was fascinated and really happy for me. It was one of the best days of my life to date! It was validation that everything out of the standard box I had intuitively sought and experimented with had worked!

I have now been in the process of reintroducing my spine to the active things that I have always enjoyed in my life: golf, tennis, jogging, strong workouts, and looking forward to wake boarding and snowboarding next year. My mission now is to get in the best physical shape that I possibly can especially around my core to assist in protecting my spine, which is very important. I am well on my way with that in addition to learning about and incorporating healing natural foods that work well with my specific makeup. I am continuing to work with my body and not against it, pushing past prior physical and mental limitations to see what I am now capable of doing, and building on that every day.

Many of the ailments we face today are often times a derivative of our own doing, lifestyles, and/or life experiences in some way shape or form that have manifested in different ways with in us. We live in such a rushed, quick fix, don't have time for this kind of society and/or we're scared to take a deep dive into ourselves, or our pasts, to seek healing from the inside out. Our bodies are designed to heal themselves and tell us what they need. It is up to us to listen, respond, and be an active participant in that response. If given the time, attention, care and space, our bodies are 100% capable of regeneration, renewal, and healing when given the chance to do so.

My purpose for myself and for you is to learn and know that there are other holistic resources and modalities of healing available to us. As unconventional as a Landmark Forum, an energy coach, Ayahuasca ceremonies in the depths of the jungle, a Buddhist Llama, clearing chakras on an around the world trip, learning and implementing meditation and breathing practices, and a stem cell procedure may sound, they were all part of my healing journey. I am certainly not saying that these modalities are right for everyone and sometimes we do actually need Western medicine. However, they indeed worked for me. Our bodies and minds combined with our spirit and sheer will are capable of extraordinary results.

About the Author

Lisa Marie Crawford

Lisa Marie Crawford was born and raised in Arizona and is the youngest of three children. She is a successful and professional career saleswoman and earned a Bachelor of Science in Business Marketing. Lisa Marie is an adventure seeker and is passionate about travel, having been to 43 countries so far.

Contact Information:

If my chapter speaks to you, please visit me on Instagram at lmc_traveljunkie for updates on my coming documentary of my full story and quest of healing. You may also email me at lisamcraw79@gmail.com for any additional questions you may have about my journey or if you would like further information on the many resources, individuals or modalities I used listed above that were not written about here. I am happy to share all that I know to help anyone I can through my shared experiences.

About the Editor

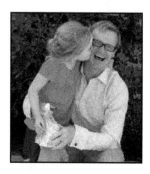

Steven E. Schmitt

Steven E has made over 1,000 books bestsellers. He can make your book a bestseller on BarnesandNoble.com, Amazon.com or even on the *New York Times* book list.

He has worked with world-renowned authors, top doctors, CEOs of major companies, top fiction and non-fiction authors, and owners of top franchises. He loves helping authors, who have a powerful message, learn how to get it out to the world.

Go to www.bestsellerguru.com for your FREE book, *How I Sold Millions of Books.*

You can find more information go to my YouTube channel:
bestsellerguru
[over 100 book marketing videos]

email Steven at:
Selawofpositivity@gmail.com

or call Steven on:
1-562-884-0062
(I will do my best to get back to you as soon as I can but remember I'm very busy with authors from around the world)

CPSIA information can be obtained
at www.ICGtesting.com
Printed in the USA
BVHW060005120920
588488BV00003B/7